T0231949

# A History of Vascular Surgery

SECOND EDITION

Always,
Heidi

# A History of Vascular Surgery

## SECOND EDITION

**Steven G. Friedman,** M.D.

Chairman, Department of Surgery
NYU Downtown Hospital
New York, New York
and
Associate Professor of Surgery
New York University Medical School
New York, New York

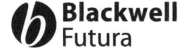

© 2005 by Futura, an imprint of Blackwell Publishing

Blackwell Publishing, Inc., 350 Main Street, Malden, Massachusetts 02148-5020, USA
Blackwell Publishing Ltd, 9600 Garsington Road, Oxford OX4 2DQ, UK
Blackwell Publishing Asia Pty Ltd, 550 Swanston Street, Carlton, Victoria 3053, Australia

02 03 04 05 5 4 3 2 1

ISBN: 1-4051-2522-5

Catalogue records for this title are available from the British Library and Library of Congress

Acquisitions: Steven Korn
Production: Julie Elliott
Typesetter: SNP Best-set Typesetter Ltd., Hong Kong


For further information on Blackwell Publishing, visit our website:
www.blackwellfutura.com
www.blackwellpublishing.com

**Notice:** The indications and dosages of all drugs in this book have been recommended in the
medical literature and conform to the practices of the general community. The medications
described do not necessarily have specific approval by the Food and Drug Administration for use
in the diseases and dosages for which they are recommended. The package insert for each drug
should be consulted for use and dosage as approved by the FDA. Because standards for usage
change, it is advisable to keep abreast of revised recommendations, particularly those concerning
new drugs.

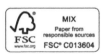

# Contents

# Foreword to first edition (abridged)

Steven Friedman approached me approximately three years ago and asked if I thought there was a need for a book devoted to the history of vascular surgery. My response, I believe, was that there is always a need for a *good* book on any subject. Before responding further, I searched my memory for any books devoted to the broad topic of vascular surgery. There was not an overwhelming number. There were some books devoted to specific areas within vascular surgery such as varicose veins, cerebrovascular disease, and peripheral arterial disease. There was only a small number of textbooks of vascular surgery. To attest to the youth of the specialty and the rapid technical changes occurring within it, there were more atlases of vascular operations than there were textbooks. The few books devoted to the history of vascular surgery were short biographies of some of its more illustrious pioneers. A few condensed histories appeared in surgical journals, usually written as a Presidential Address by one of the modern pioneers. With those thoughts in mind, I could truthfully respond to the aspiring author that there was a need for a book devoted to "A History of Vascular Surgery."

The plan for the book was to follow the progress of vascular surgery from antiquity to the present. The emphasis was to be on the accomplishments of individuals. The question of who the individual was, what he did, and the importance of his contribution was, for the most part, to be learned in the library. Whenever possible, surgeons responsible for the recent developments were to be interviewed. To accomplish this, the author read over 90 percent of the original or translated articles in his bibliography and interviewed over twenty-five contemporary vascular surgeons.

I have had the opportunity of reading the entirety of the author's contribution on two occasions. The first draft of each chapter has arrived in my office regularly every few months during a period when the author was completing his residency and establishing a practice. As residents with whom I have written papers can attest, my technique for reviewing papers is simple. I rewrite what I don't like and add some suggestions for minor changes. I next saw these chapters in the final manuscript submitted for publication. I was very impressed. I found a finished product that embodied thought-provoking quotations preceding each chapter, accurate reporting, interesting excerpts from the lives of the pioneers, and the sources of many familiar quotations. The book was of reasonable length and more than covered the highlights of the history of vascular surgery. The flavor of the author's style appeared throughout the book and none of my rewritten paragraphs were to be found.

One of the most pertinent quotations appears at the beginning of the chapter on Recent Advances. Henry L. Ellsworth, Commissioner of Patents in 1843, stated: "The advancement of the arts from year to year taxes our credulity and seems to presage the arrival of that period when human improvement must end." The incorrectness of that statement has been emphasized by the continual advances which have occurred in vascular surgery since 1843 and the realization that the Fogarty catheter, balloon angioplasty, and laser surgery are just the beginning of many more improved techniques available to the vascular surgeons of the future.

James A. DeWeese, M.D.
Professor of Surgery
Chairman Cardiothoracic Division
University of Rochester
School of Medicine and Dentistry
Rochester, New York
1989

# Foreword

Students of medical history and practitioners should take delight in reading this new edition of Steven Friedman's *A History of Vascular Surgery*. If the author was considered to be an aspiring writer with the publication of his original text in 1989, he must now be recognized as an accomplished contributor to our understanding of the historical underpinnings of one of medicine's newest disciplines – vascular surgery. A few tidbits reflect the breadth of this book.

Sushruta, a talented and productive surgeon from the subcontinent of India who lived more than 2500 years ago, is described as the first to discuss the control of bleeding vessels in a systematic manner (Chapter 1). He was also clear in his condemning those who performed the wrong operation because of mistakes or a lack of skill, as well as for greed. His statement on incompetent surgeons has become increasingly relevant in our contemporary times of greater physician accountability. The simple control of bleeding by Celsus, Antyllus, and Galen characterized vascular surgery during antiquity. More complex interventions were heralded by Richard Lambert, who was among the first to describe an actual vascular reconstruction when he reported Hallowell's 1759 approximation of the margins in an arterial wound, an observation that changed the practice of organ- and limb-threatening ligation to a reconstructive mode (Chapter 2). Nearly a century later, John Murphy performed the first successful arterial reanastomosis in 1897.

Contributions of the Scottish brothers William Hunter and the younger John, born in the early 1700s, and the Englishman Astley Cooper, born in the mid-1700s, directed the attention of clinicians to the treatment of vascular diseases other than bleeding associated with trauma (Chapters 3 and 4). All three contributed important insights into the recognition of aneurysmal disease and its treatment, albeit by simple ligature. If there was ever a story of redemption, Astley Cooper, who self-proclaimed that he "had a way with the girls," certainly would be in the forefront (Chapter 5). He was considered to be a sad rogue as a medical student and even characterized himself as an "idle rollicking, ne'er-do-well." Obviously, he redeemed himself in his later days, having been recognized as a Baron by the King of England for his contributions to the surgical sciences.

Use of autologous vein to replace or bypass diseased and injured arteries signaled the beginning of modern vascular surgery nearly 100 years ago in the publications of Alexis Carrel and Charles Guthrie (Chapter 6). Although Jose Goyanes interposed a popliteal vein in place of a popliteal aneurysm in 1906, it was four decades before the success of using reversed vein for arterial reconstructions became established, and another two decades before *in situ* reconstructions became popular in clinical practice.

Nearly two centuries passed from the days of treating aortic aneurysms by ligation to the present-day era of successful endovascular graft placement (Chapter 7). During the interim period, many vascular surgeons successfully treated aortic disease with homografts. Although the history of these last conduits was short-lived, their use led to improved operative techniques that soon thereafter made the insertion of synthetic aortic prostheses an attractive and seminal event in the evolution of vascular surgery.

The history of carotid artery surgery is remarkable if only for the centuries of overlooking the extracranial portion of this vessel as a source of emboli causing stroke (Chapter 8). It was only with the development of imaging by Egas Moniz and with Miller Fisher's autopsy study recognizing that most strokes had an embolic cause that carotid revascularization became a clinical reality. Michael DeBakey's performance of the first successful carotid endarterectomy in 1953 was not reported at that time. Instead, clinical interest in carotid artery reconstructive surgery actually evolved after the 1954 report of Felix Eastcott, George Pickering, and Charles Rob, who resected a carotid bifurcation and performed a primary reanastomosis for an obstructing arteriosclerotic lesion. Four decades passed before the efficacy of carotid endarterectomy was firmly established by the North American Symptomatic Carotid Endarterectomy Trial (NASCET) and the Asymptomatic Carotid Atherosclerosis Study (ACAS) prospective clinical trial. Similar studies will be required to define the value of catheter-based carotid artery angioplasty and stenting.

Valentine Mott was one of America's first vascular surgeons (Chapter 9). He trained for 6 months with Astley Cooper in England and then returned to New York, where, at the age of 28, he became the first Chairman of Surgery of the merged Columbia College and College of Physicians and Surgeons in 1813. Mott's legacy was in treating vessels arising from the aortic arch and terminal abdominal aorta. Just as remarkable was his death at 80, when his overall health precluded amputation of a gangrenous leg.

Successful treatment of many aneurysms became more commonplace under the aegis of Rudolph Matas (Chapter 10). This American surgeon, born in Louisiana, had lived in France and Spain before returning to his home state, where he obtained his medical degree at the age of 19 in 1880. His early work at the Charity Hospital in New Orleans provided ample opportunity to treat traumatic aneurysms. It was in this environment that he perfected the technique of aneurysmorrhaphy, which allowed maintenance of distal flow in the affected artery. Shortly after the turn of the 20th century, Matas underwent an eye enucleation for infection. Loss of binocular vision certainly did not encumber his surgical prowess. Toward the end of his career, he reported more than 600 operations for aneurysms, of which 101 were variations on aneurysmorrhaphy. It was most unfortunate that he lost his remaining eye from complications of cataract surgery, rendering him blind for the last 5 years of his life until he died at the age of 97 in 1957.

Arthur Voorhees was an example of one of vascular surgery's most important innovators. Although it is reported that he struggled in undergraduate school and medical school, he made up for his travails by recognizing the importance of an error in an experiment that he had been responsible for during his residency (Chapter 11). The appearance of a misplaced ventricular silk suture in a dog's heart suggested that implantable devices could develop nonthrombogenic surfaces, and his subsequent insertion of vinyon-N prosthetic aortic grafts followed this observation. His laboratory work and the results of grafts inserted in humans were presented in 1953, 8 years after he had graduated from medical school. This work represented a singular triumph of surgical science.

Lessons learned from the battlefield regarding vascular surgery were slow in coming (Chapter 12). Like many other marks of progress, serendipity and luck played an important role. In 1536, Ambroise Paré, having exhausted his oil supply for cauterization in the battlefield, used what he thought was a poor substitute, only to recognize a day later that this was a much more effective manner of treating vascular wounds. His use of ligatures followed. This approach continued until World War II, when the high amputation rate accompanying vascular injuries was considered to be unacceptable. This caused the Walter Reed Army Hospital Group in 1949 to consider battlefield vascular repairs. Speedy transport of patients to mobile army surgical hospital (MASH) units and the expertise of surgeons during the Korean conflict overseeing this rather radical departure from the dogma of earlier centuries allowed reconstructive surgery to replace earlier nihilistic therapies.

The history of treating venous disease is remarkable for the lack of change (Chapter 13). Socrates was the first to recommend compression bandages, and Galen suggested the excision of varicosities. All of this occurred over 15 centuries ago. The mainstay of treatment remained compression. It was not until the importance of communicating veins was recognized by John Holmans in 1916, and their interruption by Robert Linton in 1938, that treatment of venous insufficiency changed. Bypass reconstructions within the venous system were undertaken sporadically during the past 50 years, being first reported in 1952 by Palma. Under appropriate circumstances, venous reconstructive surgery, including implantation of autologous valves removed from other locations, benefits properly selected patients.

Extra-anatomic or nonanatomic reconstructions represented a major redirection in the practice of vascular surgery, being first described by Norman Freeman in 1952 and subsequently popularized by many others (Chapter 14). The first axillary femoral bypass was undertaken by William Blaisdell in 1962 as an urgent alternative to a more major procedure in a patient experiencing a myocardial infarction in the operating theater. For a brief time, an axillary femoral bypass was thought to be advantageous over direct aortic surgery. This has not proven to be the case, but clearly these alternative procedures have provided life and limb salvage in patients who could not tolerate more direct arterial reconstructive procedures.

Two groups of French vascular surgeons have made many contributions to vascular surgery. The first group includes Drs. Jaboulay, Villard, Carrel, and Leriche. These individuals, born between 1860 and 1879, made many sentinel observations that advanced vascular surgery into the next century. Mathieu Jaboulay was one of the first to evert the edges of an artery anastomosis, eliminating the thromboses that compromised earlier closures (Chapter 15). Eugène Villard, like Jaboulay, carried out many experimental canine studies and was one of the first to describe characteristic changes of veins interposed into the arterial circulation (Chapter 16). Alexis Carrel clearly defined perfection in vascular anastomoses (Chapter 17). His work with Charles Guthrie at the University of Chicago represented one of the most prolific times in the history of vessel wall replacements and was, in part, the basis for his receiving the Nobel Prize in 1912. The latter part of his life was one of bitterness, beginning with his forced retirement from the Rockefeller Institute at age 65 and insinuations that he collaborated with the Germans during World War II. Both robbed science and medicine of a brilliant mind, which would have likely continued to benefit mankind had these distractions not occurred. Lastly, René Leriche, who was a medical student when Carrel was a chief resident and who was taught by Jaboulay, wrote over 1000 papers involving surgery and physiology (Chapter 18). Although his observations, which began as early as 1923, on thrombotic occlusion of the terminal aorta carry his name, he was very reticent about supporting reconstructive arterial surgery.

The second group of French vascular surgeons included Drs. Kunlin, Dubost, and Oudot. These three individuals undertook the first successful lower extremity bypass and reconstructions of the aortoiliac segment for both aneurysmal and occlusive disease. In 1948, Jean Kunlin, who was a trainee and then an assistant to Leriche, undertook a femoral popliteal bypass with saphenous vein when Leriche was traveling outside France (Chapter 19). Kunlin subsequently presented eight similar cases that same year, and changed forever the surgical approach to profound lower extremity ischemia. Charles Dubost was the first to resect an aortic aneurysm and replace it with a homograft in 1951 (Chapter 20). The patient survived for 8 years following surgery. This accomplishment radically changed the perception of vascular surgery's potential. Dubost was an exceedingly talented surgeon who also made many contributions to the surgical treatment of heart disease, having been involved with more than 15 000 cardiac procedures and with the first in Europe to use the heart–lung machine. Jacques Oudot made important observations in the experimental laboratory regarding aortic occlusive disease and the physiologic effects of aortic clamping. He rapidly applied his knowledge to the management of aortoiliac occlusive disease by successfully treating such a patient with a bypass in 1950. This was a triumph of intellect and courage. These three French surgeons had a major impact on stimulating later advances in vascular surgery that were to emanate from the western hemisphere.

Catheter-based treatment of vascular disease has caused near cataclysmic changes in clinical practice. Three individuals, Drs. Dotter, Fogarty, and Parodi, have made seminal contributions to the new discipline of endovascular surgery. Charles Dotter deserves the title of the father of interventional radiology (Chapter 22). He completed his training and had an early academic appointment in

New York at Cornell University, before becoming Chairman of Radiology at the University of Oregon at age 32, a position he held for a further 32 years. An inadvertent recanalization of an occluded iliac artery led to the concept of percutaneous transluminal angioplasty, which he successfully performed for the first time in 1964 in a patient with lower extremity occlusive disease. Dotter was also the first to undertake intra-arterial fibrinolysis, and he was the first to describe intravascular stents. He was often characterized as a cantankerous individual who changed the practice of medicine. Thomas Fogarty is best known for the development of the balloon catheter for extracting emboli and thrombi from acutely occluded vessels (Chapter 23). It is interesting that as a resident in cardiothoracic surgery at the University of Oregon he created the first balloon catheter used for iliac artery dilation by Dotter. As an entrepreneur in bringing surgical instrumentation to the patient, Fogarty has more than 100 patents and has founded more than 40 medical companies. He has no peer in this regard. The last of the three innovators in intravascular interventions is Juan Parodi (Chapter 24). After completing a surgical residency in his home country of Argentina, he embarked on further training at the University of Illinois and at the Cleveland Clinic. Dr. Parodi conceived the idea of endovascular graft placement for the treatment of aortic aneurysms. He undertook the placement of these grafts in 53 dogs with excellent results. This achievement led to the first clinical application of the technology, when in 1990 he performed the first successful endovascular repair of an abdominal aortic aneurysm in a human. This seminal work was a direct result of Dr. Parodi's creativity and early persistence in bringing this technology to clinical practice. His accomplishment transformed the practice of vascular surgery.

This gem of a book, with its many illustrations, bibliographic references, and unique organization, details the accomplishments of many well-known individuals who have practiced vascular surgery from the times of antiquity to the present, and it offers tantalizing insights into others not readily recognized in discussions of this specialty's heritage.

James C. Stanley, M.D.
Professor of Surgery
Head, Section of Vascular Surgery
University of Michigan
Ann Arbor, MI
2004

# Preface

Since the publication of the first edition of *A History of Vascular Surgery* in 1989, vascular surgery has been transformed. Technical innovations, beginning with Parodi's seminal endovascular aneurysmorrhaphy, have rapidly accelerated the evolution of our young specialty. The major vascular societies are merging to better serve our specialty and our patients, and we are grappling with profound changes in the way we train vascular surgeons. As these events unfold, it is an opportune time to update this history of vascular surgery. To chronicle the cascading advances of the past 15 years, 6 of the 13 chapters from the first edition have been revised and 11 new chapters added. Amalgamation of these two eras revealed a common thread: the continuous presence of dauntless innovators. Whether you "caught the fever" from the first edition or missed it completely, here is your second chance.

Steven G. Friedman, M.D.
2004

PART 1

# Origins

# CHAPTER 1

# Vascular surgeons of antiquity

*It [surgery] is eternal and a source of infinite piety, imparts fame and opens the gates of Heaven to its votaries, prolongs the durations of human existence on earth, and helps men in successfully fulfilling their missions, and earning a decent competence, in life.*

(*Sushruta*)

Man has always had to face the problem of hemorrhage. Vascular surgery began with the first attempt to control a bleeding vessel. A compelling body of evidence indicates that Sushruta (Figure 1.1), the great surgeon of ancient India, first practiced ligation of blood vessels. Although Sushruta's place in historical time is debated among medical historians, most scholars of ancient Indology place it between 800 and 600 BC. Sushruta was the first great surgeon of antiquity, and his monumental treatise, *Sushruta Samhita,* was the first surgical textbook. Although the original manuscript has been lost, several translations from the Sanskrit have survived.

Sushruta divided his Samhita into six parts covering all branches of medicine, but considered surgery the first and foremost. His contributions to vascular surgery included the use of hemp fibers to tie blood vessels, application of the cautery and boiling oil to check hemorrhage, and precise instruction for the performance of amputations. Sushruta also pioneered phlebotomy as a medical treatment and described four ways of arresting hemorrhage after its use: application of astringents made from tree barks (sandhana), thickening the blood by application of severe cold (skandana), drying the wound with ashes (pachana), and cauterizing veins to make them shrink (dahana). Although it is uncertain whether Sushruta specifically used catgut ligatures, they were employed by several of the prominent Hindu surgeons who succeeded him.

Sushruta's brilliance was evidenced by his contributions to nearly every present-day field of surgery. He performed rhinoplasty, laparotomy, tonsillectomy, hernia repairs, vesicolithotomy, and anal fistulotomies, in addition to many other procedures (Figure 1.2). Sushruta may have also unwittingly inspired the first malpractice attorney with his chapter from *Samhita* concerning "defective surgical operations":

A physician (surgeon) making a wrong operation on the body of his patient either through a mistake, or through the want of necessary skill or knowledge, or out of greed, fear, nervousness, or haste, or in consequence of being spurned or abused, should be condemned as the direct cause of many new and unforeseen maladies. A patient, with any instinct of self-preservation, would do well to keep aloof from such a physician, or from one who makes a wrong or injudicious application of the cautery,

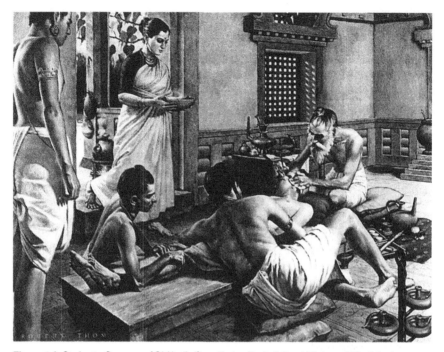

**Figure 1.1** *Sushruta, Surgeon of Old India* (from Parke, Davis & Co. *A History of Medicine in Pictures*, 1958).

and should shun his presence just as he would shun a conflagration or a cup of fatal poison.

The surgeons of Ancient Greece did not use the ligature for control of hemorrhage. They did, however, apply various mixtures of verdigris, antimony, and lead sulfate directly to bleeding wounds. A "hemostatic button," or circular wad of copper sulfate, was also used in this manner. In the fourth century BC, Hippocrates instructed that amputations be performed through the gangrenous part to avoid bleeding. When hemorrhage was encountered, however, he counseled: "Cold must be applied . . . not however to the part itself, but to the parts adjoining."

One of the earliest attempts at compiling a complete history of medicine was made by Celsus during the first century AD. Concerning the treatment of hemorrhage, Celsus advised the use of linen pledgets soaked in cold water and compressed into the wound. If this failed, vinegar was to be applied. In the worst situation, Celsus instructed that the cautery be used or that:

> . . . the bleeding vessel should be take up, and ligatures having been applied above and below the wounded part, the vessels are to be divided in the interspace that thus they may retract while their orifices remain closed.

During the second century AD, Rufus of Ephesus wrote five books of medicine. In addition to describing the importance of palpation of the pulses for

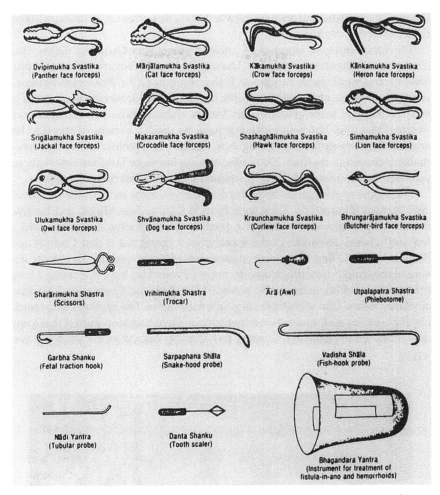

Dvipimukha Svastika
(Panther face forceps)

Mārjālamukha Svastika
(Cat face forceps)

Kākamukha Svastika
(Crow face forceps)

Kānkamukha Svastika
(Heron face forceps)

Srigālamukha Svastika
(Jackal face forceps)

Makaramukha Svastika
(Crocodile face forceps)

Shashaghālimukha Svastika
(Hawk face forceps)

Simhamukha Svastika
(Lion face forceps)

Ulukamukha Svastika
(Owl face forceps)

Shvānamukha Svastika
(Dog face forceps)

Kraunchamukha Svastika
(Curlew face forceps)

Bhrungarājamukha Svastika
(Butcher-bird face forceps)

Sharārimukha Shastra
(Scissors)

Vrihimukha Shastra
(Trocar)

Ārā (Awl)

Utpalapatra Shastra
(Phlebotome)

Garbha Shanku
(Fetal traction hook)

Sarpaphana Shāla
(Snake-hood probe)

Vadisha Shāla
(Fish-hook probe)

Nādi Yantra
(Tubular probe)

Danta Shanku
(Tooth scaler)

Bhagandara Yantra
(Instrument for treatment of
fistula-in-ano and hemorrhoids)

**Figure 1.2** Surgical instruments of Sushruta (from Prakash UBS. Sushruta of ancient India. *Surg Gynecol Obstet* 1978; 146: 263).

diagnosis, he detailed several ways to treat hemorrhage. These included compression, styptics, cautery, and twisting the arteries to occlude them. Rufus also used the ligature.

Antyllus was also a second-century physician esteemed by his contemporaries. Osler described him as one of the most daring and accomplished surgeons in history, chiefly because of his descriptions and treatment of aneurysms. Antyllus described two forms of these lesions: those originating from a local dilation in an artery, which were cylindrical, and those resulting from trauma, which were rounded. He accurately described proximal and distal ligation of aneurysms, as well as evacuation of the sac. Antyllus was ahead of his time and his treatment of aneurysms was largely forgotten until Rudolph Matas resurrected it 17 centuries later.

The most eminent surgeon of ancient Rome was Claudius Galen "the Clarissimus" (Figures 1.3 and 1.4). During the second century, he studied philosophy and medicine in Pergamon. Galen recognized the differences between arteries and veins, and devised specific techniques for achieving hemostasis in each. As surgeon to the gladiators for 3 years, Galen obtained much experience treating bleeding. For venous hemorrhage he used a variety of styptics; for arterial hemorrhage he used the ligature. Galen was a prolific writer and eventually authored more than 300 books. Among his more familiar observations was that "common sense" was a misnomer, since it was far from common.

Two aggressive surgeons of the third century were the twin brothers Cosmas and Damian (Figure 1.5). They were born in Cilicia, Asia Minor, and became famous physicians who performed great deeds of charity, never accepted a fee, and always defended Christ's teachings. Legend has it that Cosmas and Damian were the first to attempt anastomosis of blood vessels. An elderly servant of the church was afflicted with cancer of one of his legs. Following a long prayer to one of his patrons, the servant fell asleep and Cosmas and Damian appeared before him with their surgical instruments. The brothers amputated his diseased leg and remembered that a Moor slave had been buried that same day at St. Peter's cemetery. Cosmas and Damian rushed to the slave's grave,

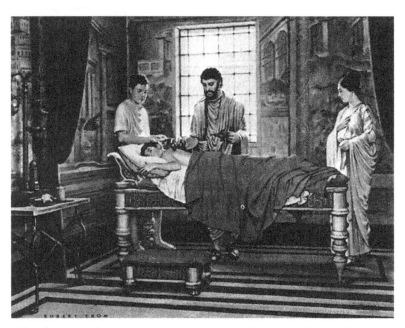

**Figure 1.3** *Galen: Influence for 45 Generations* (from Parke, Davis & Co. *A History of Medicine in Pictures*, 1958).

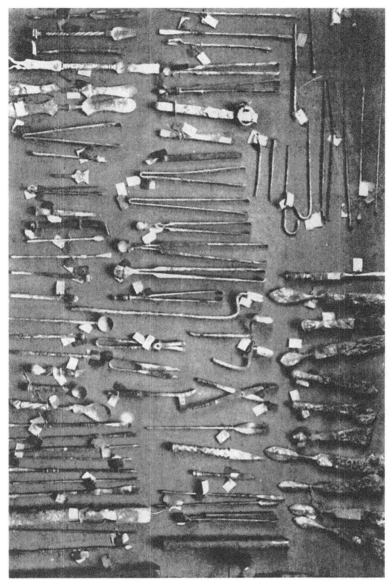

**Figure 1.4** Surgical instruments of Galen's time (from Major RA. *A History of Medicine.* Springfield, IL: Charles C Thomas, 1954).

exhumed the body, amputated the dead man's leg, and attached it to their patient's stump. The church servant awoke with one black and one white leg. Unsure of whether or not he had been dreaming, the servant went to the cemetery where the Moor's body was surrounded by a crowd of curious onlookers. Next to the slave lay the servant's diseased white leg. As a result of this and other mira-

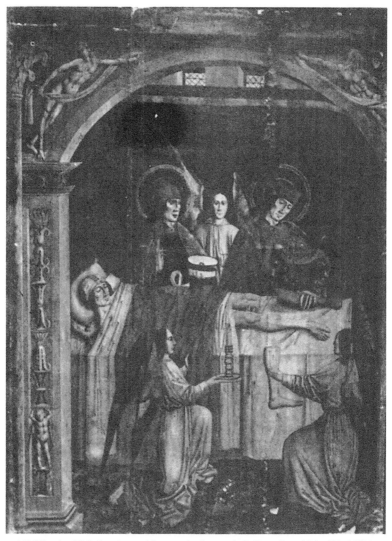

**Figure 1.5** *Miracle of S.S. Damian and Cosmas* by Fernando Gallego (from Major RA. *A History of Medicine.* Springfield, IL: Charles C Thomas, 1954).

cles, Cosmas and Damian became the Christian saints of surgery. Although there are several accounts of their deaths, the most widely accepted is that they were executed by the sword in AD 287 by the governor of Lycia, when they refused to submit to idolatry. Cosmas and Damian died martyrs and are commemorated in numerous Renaissance paintings and frescos (Figures 1.6 and 1.7).

Among the great Byzantine medical writers was Aetius, who lived in the sixth century in Amida, along the Tigris River. His works consisted of 16 books,

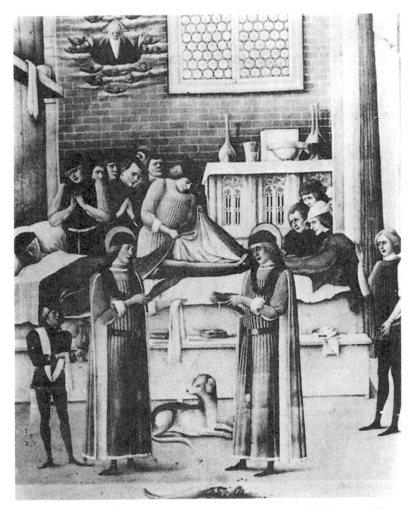

**Figure 1.6** *The Miracle of St. Cosmas and Damian* (from the School of Bellini. Courtesy of the Bettman Archive).

and in one he described the treatment of brachial artery aneurysms by proximal ligation. Aetius also was the first to ligate varicose veins.

Paulus Aegineta employed the ligature for treatment of varicose veins in a manner similar to Aetius's in the seventh century.

Albucasis of Cordova was a 10th-century Arabian surgeon who described four methods of stopping the discharge of blood from an artery: cautery, division of the artery across, use of the ligature, and styptics and bandage (Figure 1.8).

In the 11th century, Roger of Palermo employed styptics and the ligature to obtain hemostasis. He also described the "mediate ligature," a threaded needle used to suture and ligate blood vessels.

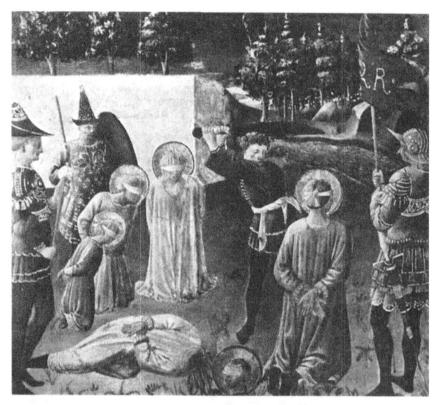

**Figure 1.7** *The Martyrdom of St. Cosmas and St. Damian* by Fra Angelico (from Castiglioni A. *A History of Medicine*. New York: Alfred A. Knopf, 1947).

The premodern history of vascular surgery concluded with the contributions of the greatest surgeon of the Renaissance, Ambroise Paré (Figure 1.9). Paré established the ligature as an effective treatment of hemorrhage. Born in Mayenne, France, in about 1510, Paré's initial training began in a barbershop and was followed by a 3-year residency at the Hotel Dieu. From 1536 to 1545, Paré acquired great experience in military surgery during the Italian campaigns. Although the ligature had been described more than two centuries earlier, Paré's greatest undertaking was reintroducing it as the preferred treatment for injured blood vessels. Paré discouraged the use of boiling oil after his supply was exhausted during a particularly fierce battle. Paré also disdained the application of a hot iron and treatment of wounds with bandages only. He was gratified to discover improved results with the ligature. In 1552, inspired by Galen's description of the ligature, Paré first used it for hemostasis. His patient was a military officer requiring lower-extremity amputation owing to wounds sustained in Damvilliers. Paré reported the case as follows:

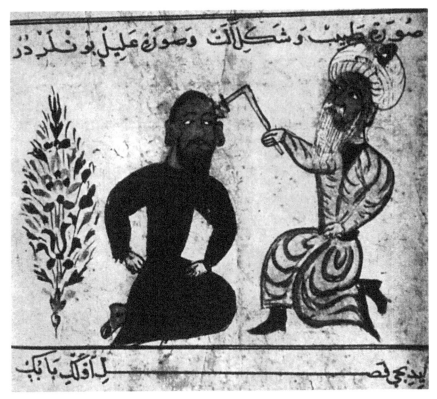

**Figure 1.8** A physician cauterizes a patient: from a 15th-century Turkish manuscript (from Castiglioni A. *A History of Medicine*. New York: Alfred A. Knopf, 1947).

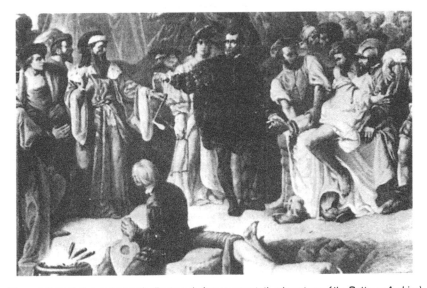

**Figure 1.9** Paré demonstrates the ligature during an amputation (courtesy of the Bettman Archive).

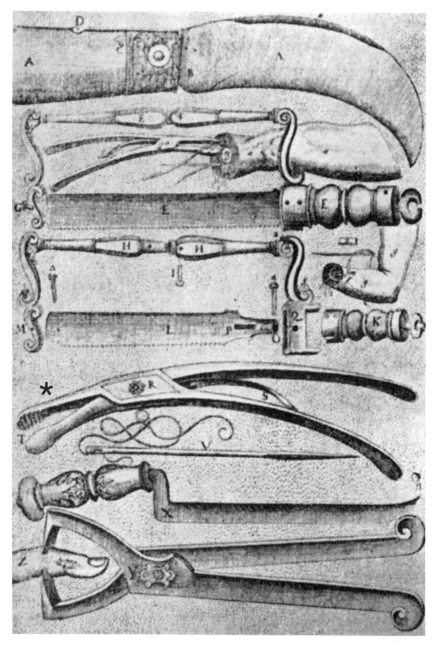

**Figure 1.10** Paré's surgical instruments. "Bec de corbin" is labeled with letters T, R, and S and is indicated by an asterisk (from Castiglioni A. *A History of Medicine*. New York: Alfred A. Knopf, 1947).

Galen wrote that it is necessary to tie the vessels toward their root, which are the liver and the heart, to staunch a great influx of blood. Having used this method of closing the veins and arteries in recent wounds several times in a case of hemorrhage, I thought that it could be done also in the removal of a limb. I conferred about this with Estienne de la Riviere, King's Surgeon-in-Ordinary, and other Sworn Surgeons of Paris, and on having disclosed my opinion to them, we decided to try it on the first patient who offered himself, keeping the cautery ready for use as did everyone else, in place of a ligature. This I have practiced thus many times with very good results, even a few days ago in the care of Pirou Garbier, a Postillion of M. Brusquet, whose right leg was removed four fingers below the knee for a mortification which had developed because of a fracture.

Paré argued vigorously for many years with his contemporaries to replace the cautery with ligation for the treatment of bleeding wounds. Paré's humility and faith in nature are epitomized by his famous remark: "I dressed him and God cured him," made after his initial use of the ligature to achieve hemostasis. Paré also observed that his patient ". . . got off cheaply without being miserably burned to stop the bleeding."

Paré introduced the first arterial forceps, his "bec de corbin" (Figure 1.10). It was originally used to extract bullets, and Paré subsequently modified it to grasp arteries to be ligated. Paré was a Renaissance surgeon. We will meet him again in the chapter concerning battlefield contributions to vascular surgery.

## Bibliography

Anning ST. The historical aspects. In: Dodd H, Cockett FB, eds. *The Pathology and Surgery of the Veins of the Lower Limb*. London: Churchill Livingstone, 1976.

Bettman OL. *A Pictorial History of Medicine*. Springfield, IL: Charles C Thomas, 1956.

Bhishagratna KLK. *An English Translation of the Sushruta Samhita Based on the Original Sanskrit Text*. Varanasi: Chowkhamba Sanskrit Series, 1963.

Castiglioni A. *A History of Medicine*. New York: Alfred A. Knopf, 1947.

Danilevicius Z. SS Cosmas and Damian. The patron saints of medicine and art. *JAMA* 1967; 2001:145.

Das S. Sushruta of India, the pioneer in the treatment of urethral stricture. *Surg Gynecol Obstet* 1983; 157:581.

Das S. Sushruta of India: Pioneer in vesicolithotomy. *Urology* 1984; 23:317.

Hamby W. *The Case Reports and Autopsy Records of Ambroise Paré*. Springfield, IL: Charles C Thomas, 1960.

Harvey SC. *The History of Hemostasis*. New York: Paul B. Hoeber, 1929.

Mukhopadhyaya G. *The Surgical Instruments of the Hindus*. Calcutta: Calcutta University, 1913.

Osler W. Remarks on arterio-venous aneurysm. *Lancet* 1915; 1:949.

Prakash UBS. Sushruta of ancient India. *Surg Gynecol Obstet* 1978; 146:263.

Southgate MT. The cover. *JAMA* 1987; 258:2630.

Toledo-Pereyra LH. A surgeon of antiquity. *Surg Gynecol Obstet* 1974; 138:767.

Tosatti B. Transplantation and reimplantation in the arts. *Surgery* 1974; 75:389.

Warren JC. *The Healing of Arteries After Ligature in Man and Animals*. New York: William Wood Co, 1886.

Zimmerman IM, Veith I. The healing saints: Cosmas and Damian. *Mod Med* 1960; 28:212.

# CHAPTER 2

# Early vascular repairs and anastomoses

*The extraordinarily delicate technic of vascular suturing is an art acquired only with much practice. It is a chapter in the history of surgery of which our colleagues may be proud.*

(Sir William Osler)

During the first half of the 18th century, chemical styptic remained the preferred treatment of bleeding vessels. Cauterization was still in use and the ligature was employed almost exclusively for controlling large vessels during amputations. Considering how little progress had been made in vascular surgery since Sushruta's work, the events of June 15, 1759, were remarkable.

Richard Lambert, a surgeon of Newcastle-upon-Tyne in England, had witnessed several cases of postoperative hemorrhage following arterial ligation, caused by erosion of the ligature through the blood vessel. Lambert had also been impressed by the functional impairment that occurred in some patients following treatment of an aneurysm by proximal and distal ligation. Physicians of the day were frequently asked to see patients with brachial artery injuries resulting from the common employment of phlebotomy to treat a variety of maladies. The occasional errant needle of the blood-letter would result in arterial laceration, false aneurysm, or an arterial–venous fistula. While examining one patient who had suffered a traumatic brachial artery aneurysm secondary to this procedure, Lambert encouraged his colleague, Hallowell, to attempt repair of the vessel without compromising the lumen (Figure 2.1). The details of this procedure appeared in a letter written by Lambert to William Hunter. Mindful of the consequences of ligating these vessels, Lambert stated:

> This case, in particular, made me turn my mind to the operation for the aneurysm, and made me wish to see it done with some alterations of the method, so as to make less disturbance in the circulation of the part.

He was hopeful that ". . . a suture of the wound in the artery might be successful; and if so, it would certainly be preferable to tying up the trunk of the vessel."

Hallowell used a half-inch steel pin to elevate the edges of the lacerated artery and tied a figure-of-eight stitch about it, thereby coapting the arterial walls. Despite a postoperative wound infection, the pin and suture were eventually extruded and the patient retained a viable extremity with a palpable pulse at the wrist. This was the first lateral arteriorrhaphy. Following the procedure Lambert contended:

> The case of the aneurysm was indeed curious, and, I am in hopes, will prove useful; but I must not be too sanguine in its favour, till I have seen the effects of such an operation confirmed by several instances; till then, I would not be fond of saying any thing of it in

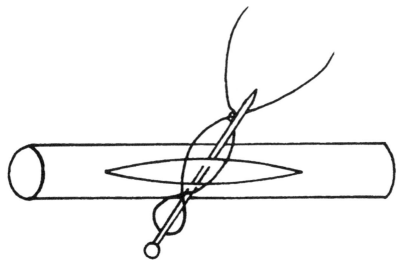

**Figure 2.1** Hallowell's arterial repair.

print, except you think, that as few of these injuries fall to any single man's share in the ordinary course of business, it would, by that means, afford a larger field to put others upon the trial, so as to introduce the method sooner.

This milestone would have gone unrecognized had William Hunter not urged Lambert to describe the operation. Lambert speculated that, if experience showed that large arteries could be repaired by placing nonobliterating sutures, the result would be an important surgical innovation:

It would make the operation for the aneurysm still more successful in the arm, when the main trunk is wounded; and by this method, perhaps, we might be able to cure the wounds of some arteries that would otherwise require amputation, or be altogether incurable.

Nevertheless, arteriorrhaphy would not gain favor until more than a century later owing to the discouraging results of experiments conducted by Assmann of Groningen. He attempted to repair lacerations in canine femoral arteries but abandoned these efforts after the first few resulted in thrombosis. Assmann concluded that the method was effective in stopping hemorrhage, but any irritation of a blood vessel resulted in immediate thrombosis. Operative repair of arteries with preservation of the lumen was therefore not possible. Unfortunately, Assmann's statements, which were based on four unsuccessful experiments, were widely accepted. Further attempts at arterial repair would not take place until the latter part of the 19th century.

The possibility that a laceration in a vein is amenable to suture repair was first suggested by Gensoul in 1833. Several experiments carried out on horses, however, resulted in venous thrombosis.

In 1843, Wattman utilized forceps to hold up the injured portion of a vein and place a ligature about it.

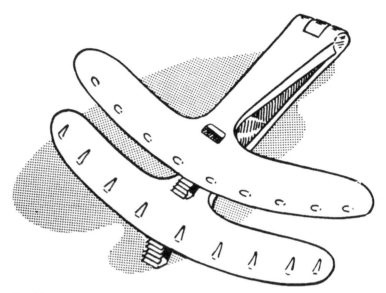

**Figure 2.2** Gluck's ivory clamp (from Callow AD. Historical development of vascular grafts. In: Sawyer PN, Kaplitt MJ, eds. *Vascular Grafts*. New York: Appleton-Century-Crofts, 1978).

In 1872, Nicaise wrote that lateral venorrhaphy was possible, and referred to the work of Gensoul.

These early attempts at vascular repair frequently met with failure owing to the inevitable development of sepsis; however, they laid the groundwork for the flurry of experimentation in vascular surgery that would soon take place. More widespread success in repairing vascular injuries awaited the contributions of Joseph Lister.

In 1867, Lister's paper on antisepsis in surgery appeared in *The Lancet*. The first vascular surgeon to adhere to the principles outlined by Lister was Czerny, who, in 1881, during an esophagotomy for removal of a foreign body, repaired a venous injury under aseptic conditions. His patient, however, succumbed to postoperative sepsis.

The following year, Gluck successfully repaired an arterial wound in the femoral artery of a dog with the aid of a small ivory clamp (Figure 2.2). All of Gluck's previous experiments had failed owing to his inability to control suture line bleeding.

A landmark development in the history of vascular surgery occurred in 1877, in Pavlov's laboratory in Leningrad. Nikolai Eck was studying the effects of directing blood flow away from the liver. Following experiments in more than 60 dogs, he devised the first portacaval shunt, or Eck fistula. Eck used a continuous silk suture to anastomose the two veins, then he opened them blindly, using a pair of scissors that had been modified for this purpose. Although Eck had little interest in vascular surgery, he performed the first documented anastomosis of two blood vessels. Eck was forced to end his research in order to join the army, and his contribution was forgotten for many years.

The first successful repair of a venous laceration was effected by Schede in 1882. He also encouraged other surgeons to use lateral venorrhaphy for civilian and intraoperative traumatic venous injuries.

Alexander Jassinowsky of Dorpat deserves the credit for first demonstrating that injured arteries could be repaired with preservation of patency. He published the results of his experiments in 1889 in his inaugural dissertation.

Jassinowsky performed longitudinal and transverse arteriotomies and then sutured them closed in the carotids of large dogs, horses, and calves. He used fine curved needles and fine silk, placed his sutures 1 mm apart through the adventitia and media only, and stressed asepsis. Of 26 experiments, 22 were successful. Jassinowsky examined his specimens up to 100 days later and reported no secondary hemorrhage, thrombosis, or aneurysm formation in the successful cases.

In 1890, Burci repeated Jassinowsky's work in dogs and horses. He substituted a continuous suture technique and reported success in four of six experiments.

Just prior to the end of the 19th century, several surgeons in different regions began experimenting with the use of rigid prostheses to reapproximate divided arteries. The first of these was Robert Abbe, a New York surgeon, who performed experiments on the femoral arteries of dogs and the aorta of a cat. After dividing these vessels, he placed thin, half-inch glass tubes, shaped like an hourglass, within the proximal and distal lumens. He then reunited the vessels over the prosthesis with fine silk. The canine femoral prostheses thrombosed, but the tube placed into a feline aorta remained patent. Abbe reported his results at a surgical conference in 1894:

> The cat made a perfect recovery, and after four months I show you him tonight, fat and strong, with a glass tube in his aorta.

This was the first experimental restoration of arterial continuity with a prosthesis (Figure 2.3).

Queirolo and Masini also performed end-to-end anastomoses over glass tubes, with a modification to Abbe's technique. Following placement of the tube, they rolled back the edge of one of the arterial segments and invaginated it within the second segment. The two vessels were then held together by a circumferential ligature. Queirolo and Masini reported their method in 1895.

Prostheses made of materials other than glass were also used in attempts to bridge injured or divided vessels. In 1897, Nitze used ivory tubes and an invagination technique similar to that of Queirolo and Masini.

An appliance which gained a great deal of attention for several years was made of small magnesium tubes and introduced by Erwin Payr in 1900 (Figure 2.4). Payr held divided blood vessels together over his prosthesis with separate

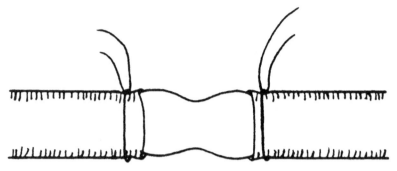

**Figure 2.3** The hourglass prosthesis of Abbe.

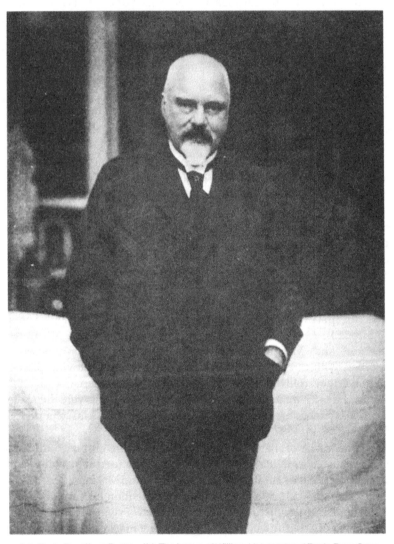

**Figure 2.4** Erwin Payr (from Rutkow IM. The letters of William Halstead and Erwin Payr. *Surg Gynecol Obstet* 1985; 161:75; reprinted by permission).

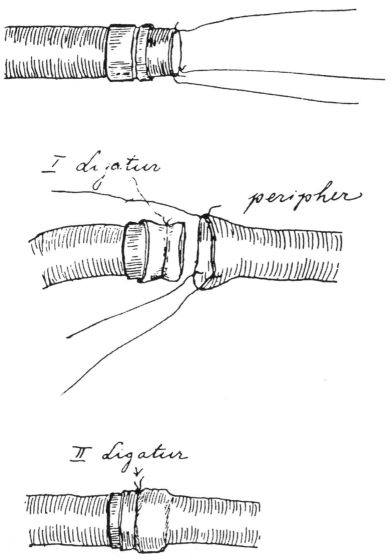

**Figure 2.5** Payr's illustration of the use of magnesium tubes (from Payr E. Weitere mittheilungen ueber verwendung des magnesiums bei der naht der blutgefaessen. *Arch Klin Chir* 1901; 64:726).

ligatures about each end of the vessel (Figure 2.5). Payr assumed that, since magnesium is soluble *in vivo*, a patent lumen would result. He utilized this technique in 1901, following resection of a groin tumor with a segment of the femoral vein to which it had become adherent. Payr bridged the resulting venous gap with one of his magnesium tubes. When the patient died three days later of pneumonia, the prosthesis was patent.

Numerous subsequent experiments in several different laboratories revealed that Payr's tubes inevitably resulted in thrombosis and could not be used clinically. Undaunted, Payr later added disk flanges to his tubes in an attempt to improve them.

In 1903, Hoepfner modified Payr's technique by using magnesium rings as collars around the divided vessels and everting the arterial edges over them. He would then join the collars together with sutures and special holding devices. Hoepfner attempted the transplantation of canine limbs with this technique, with limited success.

Even Alexis Carrel sought the ideal rigid arterial prosthesis for several years while in France. He experimented with caramel stents which were supposed to dissolve like Payr's magnesium tubes, leaving behind a patent lumen. These too were unsuccessful.

Recent attempts at arterial anastomosis with various adhesive agents descend from the work of George Brewer. In 1904, he reported in the *Annals of Surgery* his experimental attempts at closure of wounds of larger arteries with strips of aseptic, elastic plaster (Figure 2.6).

Several years later, Breer and Leggert used glass tubes lined with paraffin to rejoin arteries. In 1908, Ward attempted blood vessel anastomoses with rubber tubing.

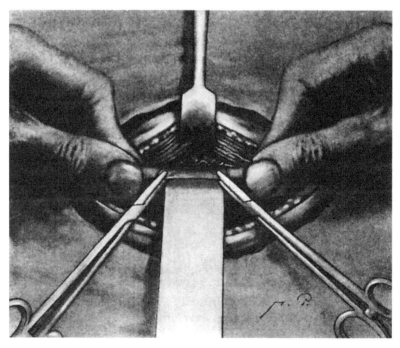

**Figure 2.6** Elastic plaster used by Brewer for arterial repair (from Brewer GE. Some experiments with a new method of closing wounds of the larger arteries. *Ann Surg* 1904; 40:856).

While surgeons around the world experimented with various materials from which rigid tubes could be fashioned and placed in the arterial tree, others continued to evaluate new sutures and techniques for repair or anastomosis of blood vessels. A notable contributor was John Murphy of Chicago, who was familiar with the work of Gluck and Jassinowsky (Figure 2.7). Murphy performed end-to-end anastomoses of canine and calf aortas, carotid arteries, and femoral arteries in 34 experiments. Murphy invaginated one cut arterial end into another, in an end-to-end fashion, and used partial-thickness sutures to hold them in place. In addition to silk, Murphy also utilized kangaroo tendon for suture.

On October 7, 1896, Murphy operated upon a 29-year-old peddler who had been shot in the groin and had developed a false aneurysm. Using his invagination technique, Murphy resected the damaged portion of the common femoral artery and reunited the vessel. The patient recovered, with an intact circulation. This was the first successful case of an end-to-end arterial anastomosis. Murphy reported his techniques and results in the *Medical Record* in 1897; his method gained popularity owing to the relative ease with which anastomoses could be performed. Murphy's work was a major step in establishing the superiority of suture repair to ligation for arterial wounds (Figure 2.8).

One year earlier in France, Mathieu Jaboulay had reported his successful attempts at reuniting the carotid arteries of donkeys and dogs. Working with Briau, he used mattress sutures to achieve eversion and approximation of the intima of both vessels. This was an important contribution since it stressed accurate approximation of all layers of the blood vessel wall. Jaboulay and Briau used interrupted U-shaped sutures and also described interposition of carotid segments into the contralateral carotid artery. In 1898, they presented a specimen to the Medical Society of Lyons that demonstrated perfect endothelial union with no thrombus formation. Jaboulay's technique would soon be improved by one of his pupils, Alexis Carrel (Figure 2.9).

Julius Doerfler, like Jaboulay, demonstrated that inclusion of the intima in an arterial suture did not necessarily lead to thrombosis. He used fine silk on curved, round needles to perform his anastomoses. Adhering strictly to aseptic technique, Doerfler reported patent anastomoses following 12 of 16 experiments in 1899. Working without any apparent knowledge of Jaboulay's contributions, Salomoni developed a similar technique in 1900.

One year later, Bougle described a modification of John Murphy's invagination method of anastomosis, in which traction sutures were placed in the leading edge of the intussusceptum and then additional sutures along the margin of the intussuscipiens (Figure 2.10).

At the turn of the century, many workers were involved in a search for the ideal method to suture blood vessels. In 1894, Heidenhain used catgut sutures to successfully repair an axillary artery laceration during excision of a carcinoma. The following year he reported the use of continuous catgut sutures and intima-to-intima reapproximation in his experiments on canine femoral and carotid arteries. Heidenhain used full-thickness sutures, and his procedures all resulted in thrombosis.

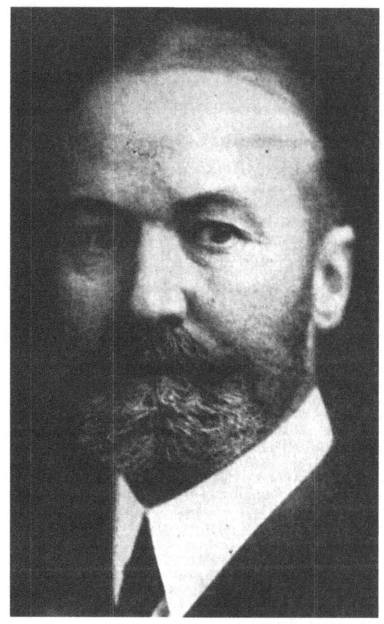

**Figure 2.7** John B. Murphy (from Major RA. *A History of Medicine.* Springfield, IL: Charles C Thomas, 1954).

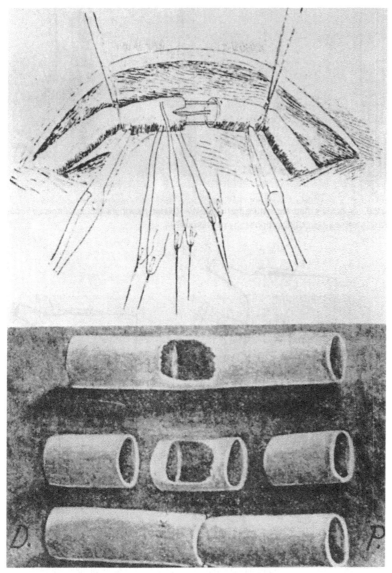

**Figure 2.8** Murphy's illustrations of the technique used for the first successful clinical end-to-end arterial anastomosis (from Murphy JB. Resection of arteries and veins injured in continuity – end-to-end suture – experimental and clinical research. *Med Rec* 1897; 51:73).

Von Horoch experienced a similar lack of success in his attempts to reunite severed arteries a few years earlier, and wrote disparagingly of this possibility.

In 1901, Clermont described the use of the whip stitch to try to limit suture-line bleeding. He would backtrack after several sutures to reinforce the anastomosis. George Dorrance also used this backtrack technique, in addi-

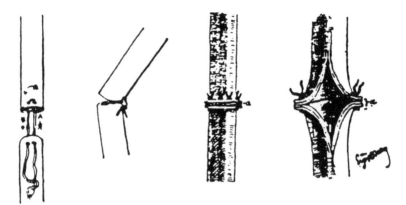

**Figure 2.9** Jaboulay's mattress suture (from Dale WA. *Management of Vascular Surgical Problems*. New York: McGraw-Hill, 1985; reprinted by permission).

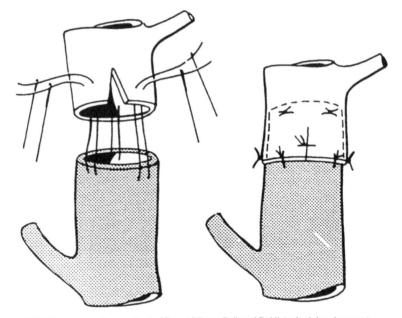

**Figure 2.10** The invagination method of Bouglé (from Callow AD. Historical development of vascular grafts. In: Sawyer PN, Kaplitt MJ, eds. *Vascular Grafts*. New York: Appleton-Century-Crofts, 1978).

tion to continuing the original suture back over the first layer with a whip stitch to prevent anastomotic leaks. He reported this technique in the *Annals of Surgery* in 1906 (Figure 2.11).

The experimentation in vascular surgery throughout the world at the beginning of the 20th century demonstrated that the field was in its infancy, led by

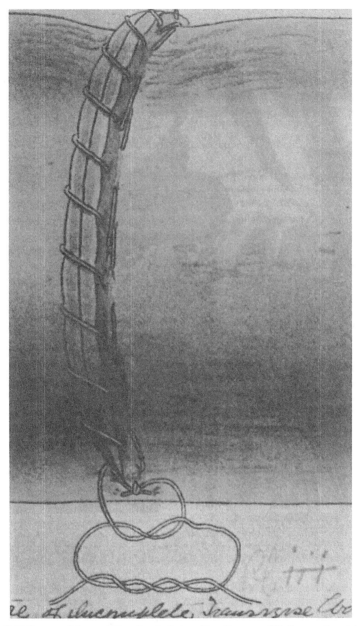

**Figure 2.11** Dorrance's hemostatic suture technique (from Dorrance GM. An experimental study of suture of arteries with a description of new suture. *Ann Surg* 1906; 44:409).

many individuals with little or no experience. No consensus of opinion existed regarding either the correct way to reunite blood vessels (directly or with prostheses) or the choice of an appropriate suture technique. Many techniques were purported to be the best, yet all remained unproven. The stage was set for one individual to evaluate and correct the wealth of conflicting data, and to set the infant field of vascular surgery on the road to maturity. We will meet Alexis Carrel in "The French connection."

## Bibliography

Abbe R. The surgery of the hand. *NY Med J* 1894; 59:33.

Bouglé. La suture artérielle, étude critique et expérimental. *Arch Med Exp D'Anat Path* 1901; 13:205.

Brewer GE. Some experiments with a new method of closing wounds of the larger arteries. *Ann Surg* 1904; 40:856.

Burci E. Ricerche sperimentali sul processo di riparazione delle ferite longitudinali delle arterie. *Zentr Chir* 1890; 17:897.

Callow AD. Historical development of vascular grafts. In: Sawyer PN, Kaplitt MJ, eds. *Vascular Grafts*. New York: Appleton-Century-Crofts, 1978.

Carrel A. La technique opératoire des anastomoses vasculaires et de la transplantation des viscères. *Lyon Med* 1902; 98:850.

Child CG. Eck's fistula. *Surg Gynecol Obstet* 1953; 96:375.

Clermont G. Suture laterale et circulaire des veines. *Presse Med* 1901; 9:229.

Doerfler J. Ueber arteriennaht. *Beitr Chir* 1899; 25:781.

Dorrance GM. An experimental study of suture of arteries with a description of new suture. *Ann Surg* 1906; 44:409.

Ehrenfried A, Boothby WM. The technic of end-to-end arterial anastomosis. *Ann Surg* 1911; 54:485.

Guthrie CC. *Blood Vessel Surgery and Its Applications*. London: Longmans Green, 1912.

Heidenhain L. Ueber naht von arterienwunden. *Zentr Chir* 1895; 49:1113.

Hoepfner E. Ueber gefaessnaht, gefaesstransplantationen und replantation von amputirten extremitaeten. *Arch Klin Chir* 1903; 70:417.

Jaboulay M, Briau E. Recherches expérimentales sur la suture et la greffe artérielle. *Lyon Med* 1896; 81:97.

Kummell H. Ueber circulaere gefaessnaht beim menschen. *Beitr Klin Chir* 1900; 26:128.

Lambert. Extract of a letter from Mr. Lambert, surgeon at Newcastle upon Tyne, to Dr. Hunter; giving an account of a new method of treating an aneurysm. Read June 15, 1761. *Med Obs Inq* 1762; 2:360.

Matas R. Vascular surgery. In: Keen WW, DaCosta JC, eds. *Surgery, its Principles and Practice*. Philadelphia: WB Saunders, 1911.

Murphy JB. Resection of arteries and veins injured in continuity – end-to-end suture – experimental and clinical research. *Med Rec* 1897; 51:73.

Payr E. Zur frage der circulaeren vereinigung von blutgefaessen mit resorbirbaren prothesen. *Arch Klin Chir* 1900; 62:67.

Payr E. Weitere mittheilungen ueber verwendung des magnesiums bei der naht der blutgefaessen. *Arch Klin Chir* 1901; 64:726.

Schede M. Einige bemerkungen ueber die naht von venenwunden, nebst mittheilung eines falles von geheilter naht der vena cava inferior. *Arch Klin Chir* 1892; 43:338.

Smith EA. *Suture of Arteries: An Experimental Research*. London: Oxford University Press, 1909.

Ward W. Blood vessel anastomosis by means of rubber tubing. *NY Med Rec* 1908; 74:671.

Watts SH. The suture of blood vessels. Implantation and transplantation of vessels and organs. An historical and experimental study. *Bull Johns Hopkins Hosp* 1907; 18:153.

# PART 2

# The British are coming

# CHAPTER 3

# William Hunter

*A sibling may be the keeper of one's identity, the only person with the keys to one's unfettered, more fundamental self.*

(*Marian Sandmaier*)

William Hunter was born near East Kilbride, Scotland, in 1718. During his grammar school years, which were not particularly noteworthy, Hunter planned to study theology. He eventually studied the arts for 5 years at the University of Glasgow.

At the age of 18, Hunter met William Cullen, a respected Glasgow physician who would figure prominently in the course of Hunter's life. From 1736 to 1739, Cullen introduced Hunter to the field of medicine.

In 1739, Hunter moved to Edinburgh, where he studied with Alexander Monro. Two years later he traveled to London, where he met two well-known Scottish physicians: William Smellie and James Douglas. It was under the tutelage of Douglas that William Hunter developed the approach to science and medicine for which he would become famous. He assisted Douglas in the dissecting room and attended pathology classes at St George's Hospital (Figure 3.1).

Hunter's first publication dealt with the structure and diseases of articular cartilages. His breadth of interest and fame as a teacher grew, and in 1746 he was elected to the Society of Naval Surgeons at Guy's Hospital. The following year he was inducted into the Corporation of Surgeons, and in 1750 he was awarded the degree of Doctor of Medicine from the University of Glasgow.

During his study of anatomy and pathology at St George's Hospital, Hunter was upset by the inadequacies of the medical education system. This led him to open his first school of anatomy in Covent Garden, London. In 1768, he opened a school for which he became even more renowned: the Great Windmill Street School of Anatomy. William Hunter's younger brother, John, had already joined him by 1748; together they performed many dissections on a variety of animals and specimens in the two schools (Figure 3.2).

The contribution to vascular surgery for which William Hunter is best known, and of which he was most proud, was his identification of the arterial–venous communication as an atypical aneurysm. After extensive research, he also claimed credit for its original description. Venesection was still a common practice during Hunter's time, and it afforded physicians of the day ample experience with false aneurysms and arterial–venous communications. A laboratory assistant at the Middlesex Hospital presented Hunter with one of his first cases of "aneurysmal varix," caused by the errant needle of a phle-

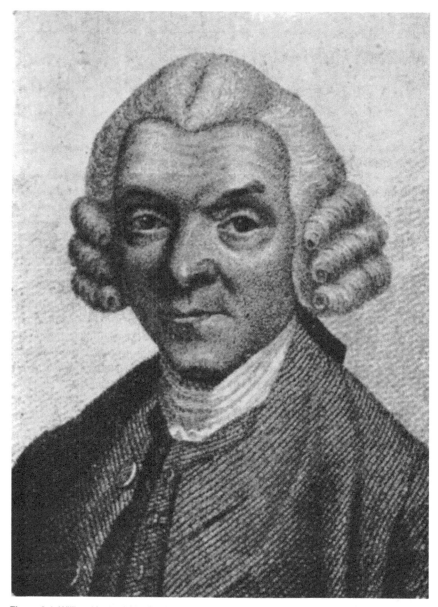

**Figure 3.1** William Hunter (from Garrison FH. *History of Medicine*. Philadelphia: WB Saunders Co. 1929).

botomist. Hunter described the veins in these lesions as being dilated or varicose, with a "pulsatile jarring" motion caused by arterial flow. He described "a hissing noise" as well, which corresponded to the patient's pulse, characteristic of a continuous bruit.

Hunter distinguished between the different approaches to the treatment of

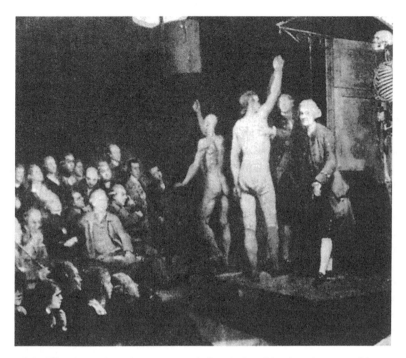

**Figure 3.2** William Hunter lecturing on anatomy before the Royal Academy (courtesy of the Bettman Archive).

aneurysms and aneurysmal varices. He stated that, because of the resistance of true aneurysms to arterial blood, they grew continuously and would burst without surgical cure. The arterial–venous communication, on the other hand, achieved a "nearly permanent state." Hunter did not recognize that these too could result in complications if untreated. Based on these observations, the ligature became the accepted treatment for true aneurysms, while arterial–venous communications were observed.

Another of William Hunter's noteworthy contributions to vascular surgery was his paper written in 1757 entitled: "The History of an Aneurysm of the Aorta with Some Remarks on Aneurysms in General." Hunter's interest in aneurysm formation began during his studies with James Douglas, who in turn subscribed to the theories of Galen.

Aneurysms were classified as either true or false and to these Hunter added a third type, which he called "mixed." These aneurysms were caused, he maintained, ". . . by a wound or rupture of some of the coats of the artery, and partly by dilation of the rest." In his treatise on aneurysms, Hunter also presented several cases of true aneurysms. Of these he said:

The spontaneous aneurysm wherever seeded is much more to be dreaded in its consequences, than one that is the immediate result of external injury. In the one, the disease is local; in the other, probably universal.

This represents one of the earliest suggestions that aneurysms could have a systemic etiology.

Reference has been made in the preceding chapter to what may have been William Hunter's greatest service to medicine, when he urged Lambert and Hallowell to report their repair of a lacerated brachial artery. In 1761, 2 years after the first successful anteriorrhaphy, Hunter reported the event to the prestigious Society of Physicians. The report was eventually published in 1762, in *Medical Observations and Inquiries*. If William Hunter had not recognized its significance, this historic event would have gone unrecorded given Lambert's modesty. Although the technique was not immediately adopted, Lambert's and Hallowell's operation would stimulate the first concerted efforts, more than a century later, to repair arteries.

William Hunter became Professor of Anatomy at the Royal Academy of Arts in 1768, and was eventually elected its president. In addition to lecturing in anatomy and surgery, Hunter also taught obstetrics. In 1774, he published one of his greatest works: *The Anatomy of the Human Gravid Uterus*.

Hunter was a tireless worker, totally devoted to medicine, and he continued to teach until his death in 1783. By that time, he had amassed a sizeable fortune, most of which he bequeathed to the Anatomical Museum at Glasgow and to the cause and progress of medical science.

## Bibliography

Beekman F. Studies in aneurysm by William and John Hunter. *Ann Hist Med* 1936; 8:124.

Chitwood WR Jr. John and William Hunter on aneurysms. *Arch Surg* 1977; 112:829.

Garrison FH. *History of Medicine*. Philadelphia: WB Saunders Co., 1929.

Illingworth C. *The Story of William Hunter*. Edinburgh: E & S Livingstone, 1967.

Osler W. Remarks on arterio-venous aneurysm. *Lancet* 1915; 1:949.

Wangsteen OH. The stomach since the Hunters. *Lancet* 1963; 83:262.

# CHAPTER 4

# John Hunter

*For faithful life-long study of science you will find no better example than John Hunter, never satisfied until he had the pericardium of Nature open and her heart throbbing naked in his hand.*

*(Oliver Wendell Holmes)*

John Hunter was born in 1728 and was 10 years William's junior. During his childhood, John received little formal education. He disliked books and was slow to read. From an early age, however, he evidenced an interest in observing nature: "I watch the ants, bees, birds, tadpoles and caddis worms; I pestered people with questions about what nobody knew or cared anything about."

At the age of 20, Hunter was still without direction and wrote to his older brother. William invited John to join him in London. From 1748 to 1751, the younger Hunter spent most of his time in his brother's Covent Garden Anatomy School. Under William's guidance, and that of the famous lithotomist William Cheselden, John became a proficient anatomist and teacher. Following the abolition of laws forbidding the practice of private dissection, the Covent Garden Anatomy School became an important center for the study of anatomy (Figure 4.1).

In 1751, John Hunter studied with Percival Pott of St Bartholomew's Hospital. In 1753, John Hunter was elected Master of Anatomy at Surgeons' Hall, and his interest spread to comparative anatomy; he acquired different animals from many sources available for dissection. From 1754 to 1756, Hunter was house-surgeon at St George's Hospital, where he made some of his greatest contributions to surgery. These included descriptions of lymphatic vessels and placental circulation.

In 1760, John Hunter joined the British Army under King Frederick and fought in Portugal during the Seven Years War. This experience laid the ground-work for his later description of the treatment of gunshot wounds. In 1794, one of his most famous works would be published: *A Treatise on Blood, Inflammation, and Gun-Shot Wounds.*

John Hunter returned to London in 1763 and commenced work on a zoo that began as a two-story, square, brick building. One can only imagine how often the house and grounds were expanded in order to accommodate the burgeoning population of birds, fish, animals, and plants that Hunter eventually collected in an attempt to capture the passion of his childhood (Figure 4.2).

In 1767, Hunter was elected Fellow of the Royal Society and a member of the Corporation of Surgeons. By this time, he had become a celebrated teacher and had helped to elevate English surgery from a technical trade to a respected pro-

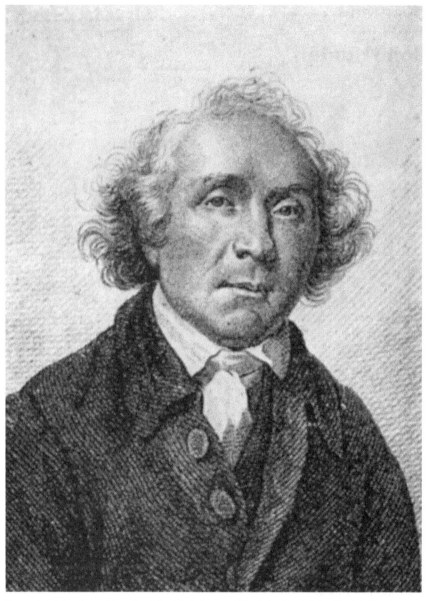

**Figure 4.1** John Hunter (from Castiglioni A. *A History of Medicine*. New York: Alfred A. Knopf, 1947).

fession. Hunter's pupils included William Blizzard, John Abernethy, Edward Jenner, and Astley Cooper. Hunter's insistence on investigation and experimentation was influential throughout the surgical communities of England and the United States.

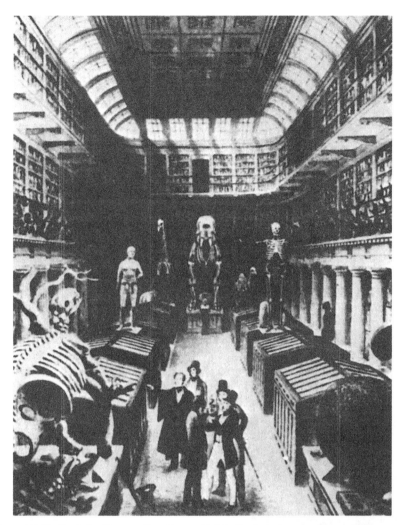

**Figure 4.2** The Hunterian Museum (from Causey G. John Hunter's museum. *Surgery* 1963; 54:692).

John Hunter is probably best known for his treatment of popliteal aneurysms, even though he did not originate it (Figure 4.3). In the 18th century, Anel, Desault, and others had ligated aneurysms of the brachial and popliteal arteries. Nevertheless, many contemporary surgeons of the time condemned the use of arterial ligation to treat these lesions, preferring instead initial amputation in light of the gangrene or exsanguinating hemorrhage that some-times resulted from ligation.

In 1779, Percival Pott stated that, no matter how judiciously performed, proximal and distal arterial ligation for aneurysm would not save the patient's

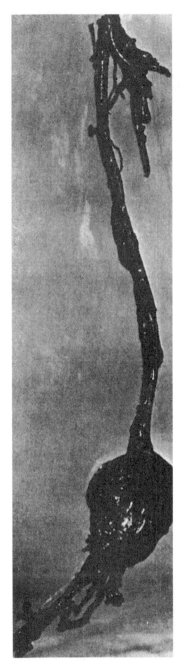

**Figure 4.3** Postmortem specimen from John Hunter's first case of ligation for a popliteal aneurysm (courtesy of the Royal College of Surgeons of England).

life. In most cases, ". . . the artery is not only dilated and burst, but it is also distempered someway above the dilatation." Hunter reasoned that placement of a proximal ligature at a distance away from the aneurysm would reduce the chances of arterial erosion. He also felt that a more remote dissection would interrupt fewer collaterals, increasing the chances of limb salvage. With this approach in mind, the stage was set for what would become his most famous operation.

Hunter's patient was a 45-year-old London coachman in whom a popliteal aneurysm had been diagnosed 3 years earlier. It had increased in size dramatically, and in December 1785 the patient was admitted to St George's Hospital. The aneurysm could easily be seen as it displaced the hamstrings on either side of it. In addition, the extremity was swollen and edematous. Hunter's brother-in-law and record keeper, Evevard Home, provided the following description of the operation, which appeared in the *London Medical Journal* 1 year later:

> Mr. Hunter having determined to perform the operation, a tourniquet was previously applied, but not tightened, that the parts might be left as much in their natural situation, as possible; and he began the operation by making an incision on the fore and inner part of the thigh rather than below its middle, which incision was continued obliquely across the lower edge of the sartorius muscle, and was made large to give room for the better performing of whatever might be necessary in the course of the operation; the fascia, which covers the artery, was then laid bare for about three inches in length, and the artery being plainly felt, a slight incision, about an inch long, was made through this fascia along the side of the vessel, and the fascia dissected off, by which means the artery was exposed. Having disengaged the artery from its lateral connexions by the knife, and from the parts behind it by means of the endave thin spatula, a double ligature was passed behind it by means of an ide probe, and the artery tied by both portions of the ligature, but so slightly as only to compress its sides together; a similar application of ligature was made a little lower; and the reason for passing four ligatures was to compress such a length of artery as might make up for the want of tightness, as he chose to avoid great pressure on the vessel at any one part.

The patient remained in St George's Hospital for 1 month and made an excellent recovery. He returned to his coach and continued to work until his death in March 1787 of "remittent fever." Hunter was present at the autopsy and, after examining the patient's lower extremity and noting that ". . . it was entirely free from putrefaction," confirmed that the operation which he had performed was unrelated to the coachman's death.

By the time of his own death in 1793, Hunter had performed the operation on four other patients, with success in three. A review of these cases was presented by Evevard Home to the Society for the Improvement of Medical and Chirurgical Knowledge in 1793. One patient survived for 50 years after Hunter's operation, and at autopsy his superficial femoral and popliteal arteries were noted to be a solid cord; the aneurysm has been reduced to a small fibrous nodule.

Hunter taught that ligation could be used for aneurysms of the subclavian, carotid, and femoral arteries as well. He cautioned that good results were dependent upon adequate collaterals and that there should be no damage to surrounding structures. Earlier operations were to be preferred before the aneurysm reached too great a size.

John Hunter's scientific pursuits spread well beyond the realm of vascular surgery. He made numerous contributions to the fields of gastric physiology, trauma surgery, and dentistry. One of his most famous publications was *The Natural History of the Human Teeth*, appearing in 1771.

It was unfortunate that Hunter's curiosity also led him to speculate on the nature of venereal disease. In May 1767, he inoculated his penis with a specimen taken from a patient suffering with urethritis. It would not be demonstrated until many years later that gonorrhea and syphilis are distinct diseases, and Hunter's inoculum also contained *Treponema pallidum*. Hunter attempted self-treatment over the ensuing years with lunar caustic and calomel, and mercurial ointment. His secondary syphilis was eventually manifested when he developed a rash and subsequent tonsillar abscess. Hunter also suffered from central nervous system complications and developed a syphilitic ascending aortic aneurysm. Toward the end of his life, John Hunter suffered frequent attacks of angina. He rued the fact that his life was ". . . in the hands of any rascal who chooses to annoy and tease me."

Hunter's description of his predicament proved accurate when, during a St George's Hospital board meeting, he was told of the appointment of his successor. His subsequent outrage resulted in a fatal attack of angina.

Through the efforts of William Clift, a great admirer of Hunter, much of his work remains today in the library of the Royal College of Surgeons in England.

## Bibliography

Beekman F. Studies in aneurysm by William and John Hunter. *Ann Hist Med* 1936; 8:124.

Causey G. John Hunter's museum. *Surgery* 1963; 54:692.

Chitwood WR Jr. John and William Hunter on aneurysms. *Arch Surg* 1977; 112:829.

Garrison FH. *History of Medicine*. Philadelphia: WB Saunders Co., 1929.

Hunter J. *A Treatise on the Blood, Inflammation, and Gun-Shot Wounds*; 1794. Birmingham: Gryphon Editions Ltd., 1982

Lasky II. John Hunter, the Shakespeare of medicine. *Surg Gynecol Obstet* 1983; 156:511.

Martin LE. John Hunter and tissue transplantation. *Surg Gynecol Obstet* 1970; 131:306.

Osler W. Remarks on arterio-venous aneurysm. *Lancet* 1915; 1:949.

Schechter DC, Bergan JJ. Popliteal aneurysm: A celebration of the bicentennial of John Hunter's operation. *Ann Vasc Surg* 1986; 1:118.

Wangsteen OH. The stomach since the Hunters. *Lancet* 1963; 83:262.

# CHAPTER 5

# Astley Cooper

*But where's the man who counsel can bestow, Still pleased to teach, and yet not proud to know?*

*(Alexander Pope)*

Astley Cooper was born in Norfolk, England, in 1768. His father was a clergy-man and his mother, a cousin of Sir Isaac Newton, was a talented writer who had inherited great wealth. Cooper's paternal grandfather was a surgeon in Norwich and his uncle William was a senior surgeon to Guy's Hospital.

Cooper was the fourth of 10 children in this distinguished family and his early lessons were ministered by his parents and the village schoolmaster. As a child, Cooper had an enormous amount of energy, none of which was devoted to his studies. He was a notorious ringleader in neighborhood gangs and constantly got into trouble. In addition, by his own confession, he "... had a way with the girls" thanks to his good looks. Cooper's family was concerned about his academic failings, except for his father who never lost faith: "There is my boy Astley. He is a sad rogue but in spite of his roguery, I have no doubt he will be a shining character."

When Cooper turned 15, it was decided that he would pursue a medical career. He was apprenticed for 1 year to Dr. Francis Turner of Great Yarmouth. In 1784, Cooper traveled to London to work with his Uncle William at Guy's Hospital. The prospect of life in London excited Astley, but his utter disregard for serious work remained unchanged and wore on the patience of his uncle. Cooper claimed to be the typical irrepressible medical student of his time, an "idle, rollicking ne'er-do-well" (Figure 5.1).

It was Mr. Henry Cline, senior surgeon to St Thomas' Hospital, who gradually harnessed and directed Cooper's reckless energy. Cooper greatly admired Cline and, after the two had spent 6 months together, Uncle William gladly relinquished all responsibility for his rambunctious nephew. Under Cline's tutelage for the next 7 years, Cooper became a good student and a great dissector. During this period, Cooper also had the opportunity to study with Dr. Munro of Edinburgh for 7 months. This was arranged to aid Cooper's recovery from typhoid fever.

In 1791, Cooper became a demonstrator in anatomy and shared lecturing duties with Cline. Two years later, he was appointed lecturer on anatomy at Surgeons' Hall, where executed criminals were dissected in public. Cooper became quite popular through these lectures and reported: "The theatre was constantly crowded and the applause excessive."

At the turn of the 19th century, William Cooper retired as senior surgeon to Guy's Hospital and his nephew succeeded him (Figure 5.2). Astley's typical day

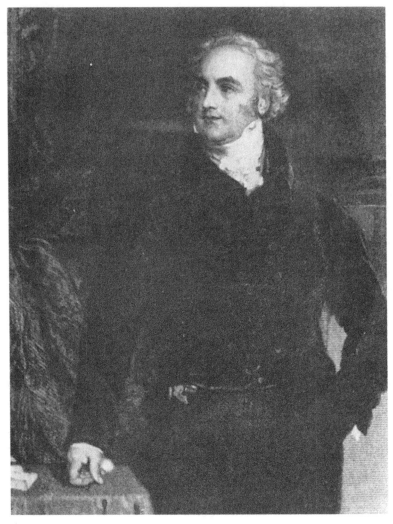

**Figure 5.1** Sir Astley Cooper (from Major RA. *A History of Medicine*. Springfield, IL: Charles C Thomas, 1954).

began at 6 o'clock, after 3–4 hours of sleep, with several hours of dissection. Following breakfast and a horseback ride, he saw charity patients for several more hours. Cooper would then ride to Guy's Hospital, where he met the medical students for ward rounds. After rounds he would perform surgery until early evening, and twice weekly he delivered 8 o'clock surgical lectures. During the night, Cooper dictated his day's activities while visiting patients in his carriage. He usually returned home at midnight, where he would read and write for several hours more. Cooper once reflected, "If I laid my head upon the pillow

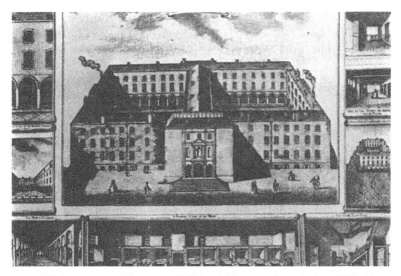

**Figure 5.2** Guy's Hospital in 1725 (from Major RA. *A History of Medicine*. Springfield, IL: Charles C Thomas, 1954).

at night without having dissected something in the day, I should think that I had lost that day."

Cooper became a Fellow of the Royal Society in 1800, where he presented his "Observations on the Membrana Tympani." Further research resulted in Cooper's discovery that some types of deafness could be relieved by myringotomy. For this he received the Copley Prize, a proud accomplishment since John Hunter had received it a decade earlier.

In 1804, the first volume of Cooper's greatest work, his treatise on hernia, was published. It wrought order out of the chaos surrounding the anatomy and treatment of hernias. The second volume appeared in 1807 and, during this time, Cooper's own umbilical and inguinal hernias were kept reduced with a truss.

Cooper eventually became known as the greatest surgical teacher in Europe. His method of systematically presenting the physiologic, pathologic, and surgical principles of diseases was unique in the early 19th century. While John Hunter laid the groundwork for surgery to become a distinct discipline based on scientific concepts, Cooper showed how these could be utilized successfully. Thousands of students throughout the world attended his lectures. Two of these included John Warren and Valentine Mott from the United States. There was one student, however, upon whom the great orations of Cooper had little effect. During one of Cooper's lectures, this particular student wrote: "The other day during the lecture, there came a sunbeam into the room, and with it a whole troop of creatures floating in the ray; and I was off with them to Oberon and fairy-land." Cooper later acknowledged that, even though young John Keats was the worst student of surgery, his poetic prowess could not be denied.

While a medical student, Cooper had studied the effects of brachial and femoral artery ligations in dogs. He had also ligated the carotid and vertebral arteries bilaterally in one animal that survived and even became "a good house dog."

In 1805, Cooper performed one of the earliest carotid artery ligations in man. Mary Edwards was 44 years old and presented to Cooper with an aneurysm of the right common carotid artery. It occupied two-thirds of her neck and the overlying skin was thin and tense. On November 1, Cooper ligated the common carotid artery of Mrs. Edwards. On November 5, Cooper found her sitting up and taking tea with some fellow patients. She appeared well except for a persistent cough. Mrs. Edwards died 16 days later and her autopsy revealed suppuration within and surrounding the large aneurysm sac, as well as compression of the larynx and trachea. Cooper concluded that the surgery would have been successful had the sac not grown so large.

Several years later, Cooper had the chance to test this conclusion when Humphrey Humphreys, a 51-year-old porter, came to see him with a left carotid artery aneurysm "the size of a walnut." On June 22, 1808, Cooper doubly ligated and divided the common carotid artery of his patient, proximal to the aneurysm. Humphreys recovered and returned to work. He survived until 1821, when he died of a left-sided cerebral hemorrhage. Cooper reported the postmortem findings in the first issue of the *Guy's Hospital Reports* in 1826 (Figure 5.3). He noted: "The disease of which he died sufficiently attested to the circulation as well as its force in the cerebral vessels on the side of which the carotid had been tied."

During the afternoon following Humphrey's operation, Cooper performed ligation of an external iliac artery for a large femoral aneurysm. This patient was a 39-year-old man from Norfolk who also recovered and lived until 1826. Cooper once remarked: "There was no man, however great or distinguished, who was likely to avoid my clutches for autopsy, as there were always means of obtaining a body you wanted." At considerable time and expense, Cooper secured the body of this patient from Norfolk and also reported his autopsy findings in the inaugural issue of *Guy's Hospital Reports*.

Cooper went on to perform external iliac artery ligation for femoral aneurysm nine more times. In 1813, Cooper was appointed Hunterian Professor of Comparative Anatomy by the Royal College of Surgeons.

The ligations of carotid and external iliac arteries were daring procedures in Cooper's time. In 1817, however, he performed his boldest operation. Charles Hutson was a 38-year-old porter who was admitted to Guy's Hospital with a large left external iliac aneurysm. It had been growing steadily for 1 year, and 3 days prior to his admission it had doubled in size. Cooper's hand was forced when the aneurysm ruptured though the skin and began bleeding. Two days earlier, Cooper had attempted retroperitoneal exposure of the aorta in a cadaver, anticipating Hutson's eventual need for surgery. He found this route "utterly impracticable" and, with Hutson in his bed, Cooper exposed the aorta through a transperitoneal incision and placed a silk ligature just above the aortic

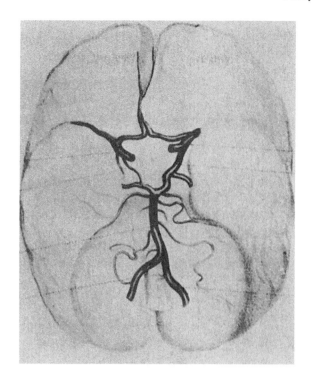

ACCOUNT

OF THE

FIRST SUCCESSFUL OPERATION,

PERFORMED ON THE COMMON CAROTID ARTERY,

FOR

ANEURISM,

IN THE YEAR 1808 : •

WITH THE POST-MORTEM EXAMINATION, IN 1821.

FROM THE NOTES OF

SIR ASTLEY COOPER, BART.

**Figure 5.3** Title page from Cooper's account of the case of Humphrey Humphreys (from Eastcott HHG. The beginning of carotid surgery. In: Bergan JJ, Yao JST, eds. *Cerebrovascular Insufficiency*. New York: Grune & Stratton, 1983; reprinted by permission).

bifurcation. Hutson appeared well the following day, but died 40 hours after surgery (Figure 5.4A and B). In his account of Astley Cooper's life, Lord Brock likened this operation to the "Everest ascent of arterial surgery of his day." Even Cooper admitted: "I was gratified when my admirers and detractors agreed

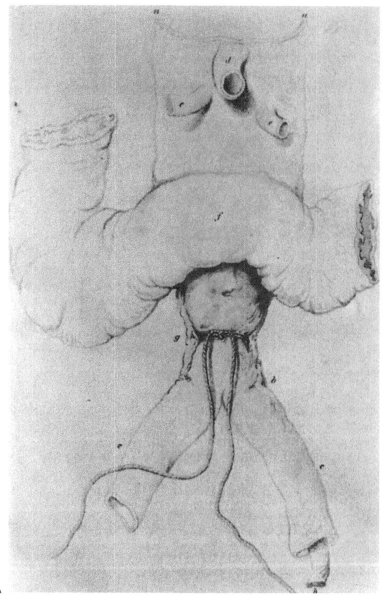

A

**Figure 5.4** Postmortem specimen from the case of Charles Hutson. (A) Anterior view; (B) posterior view (from Brock RC. *The Life and Work of Astley Cooper.* London: E & S Livingstone, Ltd, 1952).

that this was the boldest attempt to preserve life by aid of the science of surgery." Not until 1923, 106 years after Cooper's operation, would Rudolph Matas perform the first successful abdominal aortic ligation.

An additional contribution made to vascular surgery by Cooper, in 1817, was

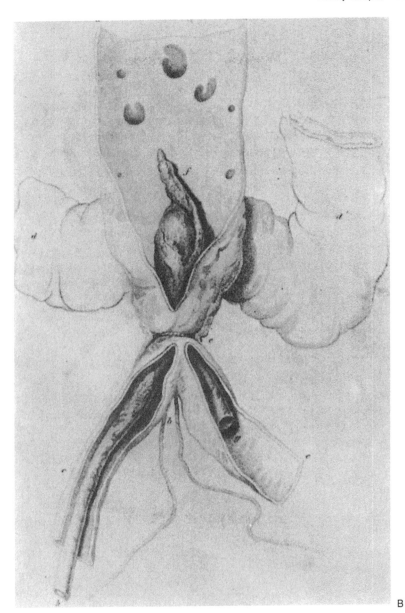

B

**Figure 5.4** *Continued*

the use of a buried catgut suture for arterial ligation. This operation on an 80-year-old man with a popliteal aneurysm was a marked departure from the usual practice of ligating the artery with silk and then bringing the ends of the ligature through the wound. This often resulted in fatal hemorrhage. Postoperative hemorrhage was avoided in Cooper's patient, whose wound was completely

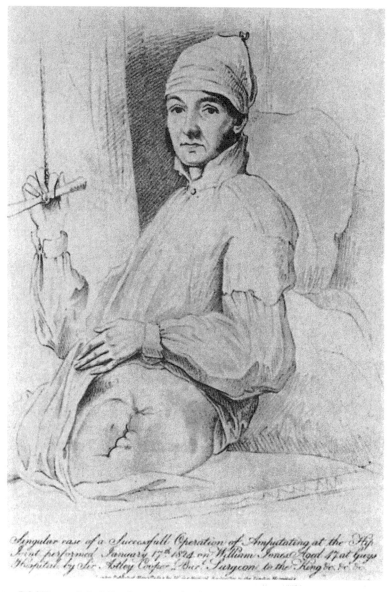

**Figure 5.5** Lithograph depicting Cooper's patient following first successful hip disarticulation (from Brock RC. *The Life and Work of Astley Cooper.* London: E & S Livingstone, Ltd, 1952).

closed over the ligature and healed without complication. Cooper remarked: "The case gave me much pleasure and the rapid recovery leads me to hope that the operation for aneurysm may become infinitely more simple."

In 1820, King George IV was suffering from an infected sebaceous cyst on his head. Cooper was summoned even though he was not one of the official Royal

Surgeons. Following excision of the cyst, Cooper described his experience briefly: "I feared erysipelas as a complication in the postoperative course of my exalted patient, but all went well and I was created Baronet by His Majesty in 1821."

In addition to his major contributions to vascular and hernia surgery, Cooper was the first to champion avoidance of amputation for compound fractures. He also offered a monograph on diseases of the testes, and a study of the anatomy of the thymus. In 1829, he published his treatise on nonmalignant diseases of the breast.

At the age of 60, Cooper relinquished his lecturing commitments because of the strain of his busy surgical practice and recurring episodes of vertigo. He was appointed an Examiner of the Royal College of Surgeons, where he assessed his fellow examiners as ". . . a doddering collection of ill-read individuals with lifetime appointments and with little interest in the welfare of the helpless candidates." This is likely the explanation of why Cooper soon became College President.

In 1840, Cooper began to suffer increasingly from dyspnea on exertion: "New Years 1841 found me in sore straights." Cooper was in congestive heart failure when he wrote those words and on February 12, 1841, surrounded by his family members and friends, his last words were: "God bless you and goodbye to you all." He was buried in a crypt beneath the chapel at Guy's Hospital.

By his own estimate, Cooper had a hand in the education of 8000 surgeons. He had an enormous surgical practice, was a master of anatomy, and displayed an unerring scientific approach to clinical problems (Figure 5.5). In the history of surgery, Cooper's contributions linked those of John Hunter and Joseph Lister. The accolade: "Prince of Surgery," bestowed upon him by his colleagues, was richly deserved.

## Bibliography

Brock RC. *The Life and Work of Astley Cooper.* London: E & S Livingstone, Ltd, 1952.

Brock RC. The life and work of Sir Astley Cooper. *Ann R Coll Surg Engl* 1969; 44:1.

Drach GW. Sir Astley Cooper (1768–1841). *Invest Urol* 1978; 16:75.

Nuland SB. Astley Cooper of Guy's Hospital. *Conn Med* 1976; 40:190.

Rawling EG. Sir Astley Paston Cooper, 1768–1841: The prince of surgery. *Can Med Ass J* 1968; 99:221.

Schoenberg DG, Schoenberg BS. Eponym: Sir Astley Paston Cooper: Good sense, good surgery, and good science. *South Med J* 1979; 72:1193.

Wass SH. Astley Cooper and the anatomy and surgery of the hernia. *Guy's Hosp Rep* 1968; 117:213.

# Divisions of vascular surgery

# Divisions of vascular surgery

# CHAPTER 6

# Development of the venous autograft

*... veins subjected to arterial flow can certainly remain intact, but have a marked tendency to thrombose when under arterial pressure. Therefore, the idea of bypassing occluded arterial pathways using neighboring veins has no practical significance.*

*(Alfred Exner)*

The first experimental attempts to place venous autografts into the arterial circulation were performed at the beginning of the 20th century by Alfred Exner, in Austria; and Alexis Carrel, in France. Exner used Payr's magnesium tubes to place canine external jugular veins into carotid arteries. The revolutionary idea of anastomosing a segment of vein directly into the arterial circulation was conceived by Carrel in 1901, at the University of Lyon. It was brought to fruition through his collaboration with Charles Guthrie at the Hull Physiological Laboratory in Chicago (Figure 6.1).

The use of metal prostheses by Exner invariably resulted in thrombosis, leading him to conclude that veins could not be used as arterial substitutes. The experiments of Carrel and Guthrie were successful owing to meticulous aseptic technique and the use of a method that did not require a foreign body other than suture material.

Carrel and Guthrie reported their canine experiments with vein grafts in a manuscript that underscored their surgical genius (Figures 6.2 and 6.3). "Uniterminal and biterminal venous transplantations" appeared in *Surgery, Gynecology and Obstetrics* in 1906. The remarks of Carrel and Guthrie regarding potential sources of vein for grafting are pertinent today:

... it is always possible to extirpate a few centimeters of vein without seriously interfering with the circulatory apparatus in general. Thus the operated subject supplies all the venous material necessary for most transplantations.

While their European colleagues were discouraged by the results of venous transplantations, Carrel and Guthrie speculated that:

The possibility of transforming a vein into an artery, from a functional point of view, naturally arouses the idea of substituting veins for arteries when the latter are rendered useless by some pathological process.

For cases of trauma or malignancy, Carrel and Guthrie wrote:

Severe subcutaneous wounds of the large arteries are ordinarily followed by serious complications, gangrene often occurring. In such cases it would be possible to extirpate freely all the injured portions of the vessel and to re-establish the circulation by interposing a segment of vein between the cut ends of the artery. The same operation would be indicated, when, during the extirpation of a large growth, the resection of an important vessel is necessary; e.g., sarcoma in the femoral region.

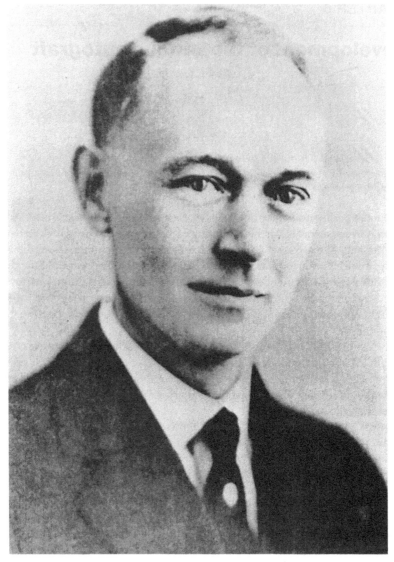

**Figure 6.1** Charles Claude Guthrie (from Callow AD. Historical development of vascular grafts. In: Sawyer PN, Kaplitt MJ, eds. *Vascular Grafts*. New York: Appleton-Century-Crofts, 1978).

The essential techniques for suturing blood vessels described by Carrel over 80 years ago are still taught to surgical residents:

> A rigid asepsis is absolutely essential for success.... The dissection of the vessel is not dangerous if the wall of the vessel is not crushed or roughly handled with metallic forceps of other hard instruments . . . it is necessary that these clamps [vascular] be smooth-jawed and not too strong in the spring . . . by using very sharp, rough needles, only extremely small wounds are made . . . great care is taken not to include fragments

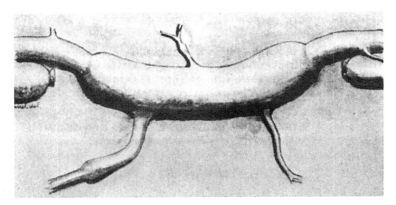

**Figure 6.2** Illustration of venous transplant into arterial circulation by Carrel and Guthrie (from Carrel A, Guthrie CC. Uniterminal and biterminal venous transplantation. *Surg Gynecol Obstet* 1906; 2:266).

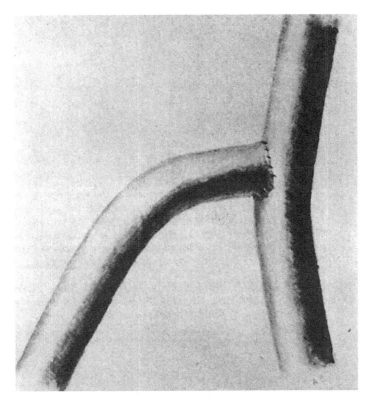

**Figure 6.3** End-to-side anastomosis of vein graft into an artery as depicted by Carrel and Guthrie (from Carrel A, Guthrie CC. Uniterminal and biterminal venous transplantation. *Surg Gynecol Obstet* 1906; 2:266).

of the connective tissue layer in the line of suturing, and to obtain a smooth union and approximation of the endothelial coats.

The first clinical anastomosis of a venous graft into the arterial circulation was performed by Jose Goyanes of Madrid (Figure 6.4). Goyanes had studied the work of Carrel, and of Murphy in the United States, and had experimented with transplantation of canine vena cava grafts into the aorta. In 1906, he was

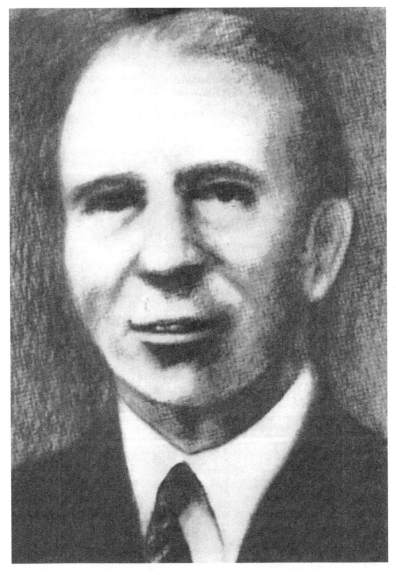

**Figure 6.4** Jose Goyanes (from Harrison LH Jr. Historical aspects in the development of venous autografts. *Ann Surg* 1976; 183:101).

asked to examine a 41-year-old candy maker who had developed a syphilitic popliteal aneurysm. On June 12, Goyanes excised the aneurysm and, unable to repair the popliteal artery primarily, used an adjacent segment of popliteal vein to bridge the defect. The patient made an excellent recovery after a postoperative wound infection, and Goyanes reported this case in *El Siglo Medico*, an obscure Spanish weekly medical bulletin. He credited his mentor, Professor San Martin, with the idea of using an autogenous vein graft in this manner. Goyanes mentioned the prior, similar use in another patient of an iliac vein segment to bypass an iliac artery obstruction. Goyanes's popliteal venous replacement of a segment of popliteal artery was also the first *in situ* vein graft (Figure 6.5).

In 1907, Stitch reported his experimental results with venous autografts. This set in motion an important chain of events. That same year, Erich Lexer of Konigsberg treated a 69-year-old man who had undergone reduction of a dislocated shoulder 9 weeks earlier (Figure 6.6). The patient had developed a large axillary pseudoaneurysm secondary to an injury to the axillary artery by the reduction procedure. Lexer had clinical experience with Payr's magnesium tube, but at surgery he was faced with an 8-cm gap between the axillary and brachial arteries after he resected the aneurysm. Lexer recognized the uselessness of a Payr tube in this situation and recalled the report of Stitch. Lexer excised a 10-cm segment of greater saphenous vein from his patient's leg and used it in a reversed manner to restore arterial continuity. Lexer's patient died of delirium tremens on the fifth postoperative day, but was found to have a patent graft at the postmortem examination which Lexer performed.

Lexer reported this case before the Congress of the German Society for Surgery, and it was published in a widely read German surgical journal: *Archives of Clinical Surgery*. Unaware of Goyanes's case the previous year, Lexer claimed to be the first to use a venous autograft to replace an artery.

William Halstead read of Lexer's case and was impressed by the report. Halstead encouraged his associate Bertram Bernheim to use venous autografts as arterial replacements in animals (Figure 6.7). Bernheim developed his vascular surgical skills in the laboratory, and in 1909 he was summoned by Halstead to apply them clinically. Halstead had removed a sarcoma from the popliteal space of a patient, resulting in a large popliteal arterial defect. Bernheim attempted to bridge the gap with a long segment of greater saphenous vein, but it thrombosed. Undaunted by this experience, Bernheim continued his laboratory research, which led to publication of a textbook on vascular surgical techniques in 1913.

Two years following publication of his book, Bernheim had a second chance to use the technique of Stitch and Lexer. His patient was a 43-year-old man with a syphilitic popliteal aneurysm. Excision of the lesion left a 15-cm gap in the popliteal artery, which Bernheim replaced with a 12-cm segment of greater saphenous vein. The patient made an uneventful recovery and Halstead praised Bernheim's efforts. This was the beginning of clinical arterial reconstruction in the United States.

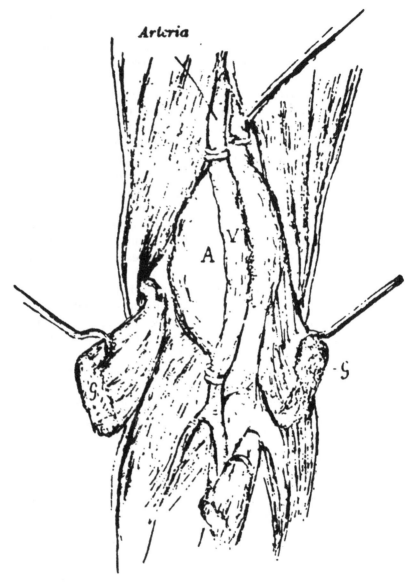

Goyanes – Madrid – 1906

**Figure 6.5** Goyanes's *in situ* bypass of a popliteal aneurysm (from Dale WA. *Management of Vascular Surgical Problems*. New York: McGraw Hill, 1985).

In 1913, Hogarth Pringle reported two cases of reversed saphenous vein grafts to maintain arterial circulation. His cases involved aneurysms of the popliteal and brachial arteries and were performed at the Royal Infirmary of Glasgow. Both operations were successful.

Further use and development of venous autografts was stimulated by

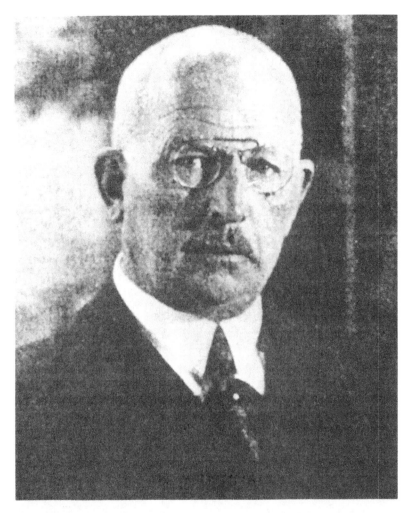

**Figure 6.6** Erich Lexer (from Harrison LH Jr. Historical aspects in the development of venous autografts. *Ann Surg* 1976; 183:101).

several contributions from other fields of science. In 1896, Wilhelm Konrad Roentgen reported his discovery of x-rays in *Nature*; 3 months later Haschek and Lindenthal performed the first arteriogram. They injected a radiopaque mixture into the arteries of an amputated arm to test Roentgen's discovery.

In 1918, Cameron reported the use of iodized salts as a contrast medium, and several years later Sicard and Forestier developed an iodized poppyseed oil called lipiodol. Sicard and Forestier performed the first clinical arteriogram when they injected their solution into the antecubital veins of a patient and observed its passage to the lungs fluoroscopically.

In 1924, Barney Brooks used injections of sodium iodide to study the arterial anatomy of the lower extremity. Great progress in arteriography was also made in Portugal, where the technique of cerebral angiography was introduced in

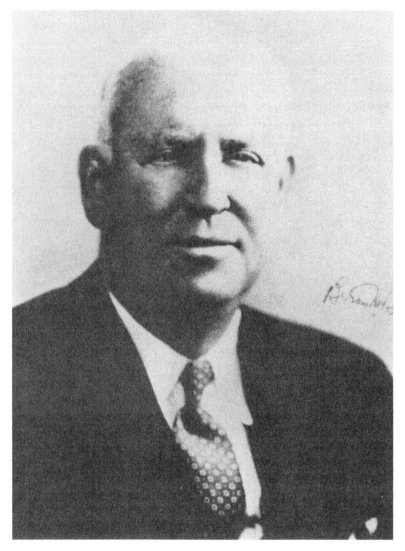

**Figure 6.7** Bertram Bernheim (from Harrison LH Jr. Historical aspects in the development of venous autografts. *Ann Surg* 1976; 183:101).

1927 by Egas Moniz. Two years later, Reynaldo Dos Santos reported angiography of the abdominal aorta, its branches, and the lower extremities (Figures 6.8 and 6.9). An accurate diagnostic procedure for vascular lesions was now available.

Little progress in vascular surgery resulted from the carnage of World War I, apart from the contributions of several German surgeons that went unnoticed. As early as 1913, Ernest Jaeger had advocated the principle of maintaining arterial continuity with various grafts, in the management of traumatic pseudo-

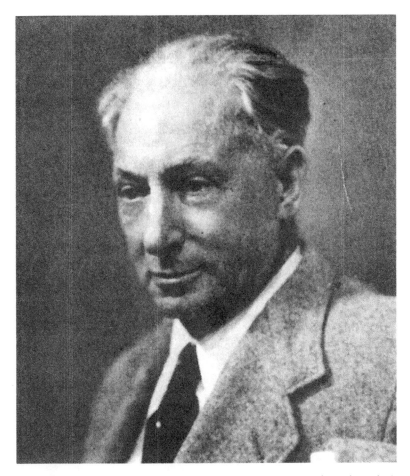

**Figure 6.8** Reynaldo Dos Santos (from Callow AD. Historical development of vascular grafts. In: Sawyer PN, Kaplitt MJ, eds. *Vascular Grafts*. New York: Appleton-Century-Crofts, 1978).

aneurysms. He later experimented with fresh venous and arterial homografts from limbs that had been severed in battle.

Warthmuller reported an 85 percent success rate in 47 cases of vein grafting for traumatic aneurysms in 1917.

Following the war, reviews by Weglowski and Lexer described 51 and 58 cases, respectively, of venous autografts for pseudoaneurysms. Lexer had one of the largest personal experiences, with 13 cases.

An important obstacle that needed to be overcome before the technique of bypass grafting could gain wider use was the problem of thrombosis. Heparin was discovered in 1916 by Jay McLean, a medical student working in the laboratory of W.H. Howell. The discovery was reported in 1918, but heparin remained too toxic for clinical use.

Best and Scott described the purification of heparin in 1933, and 5 years later

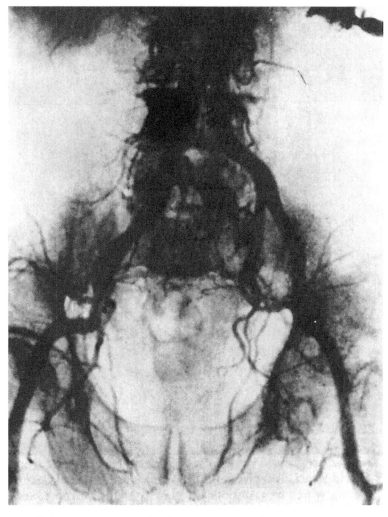

**Figure 6.9** Early angiogram performed by Reynaldo Dos Santos (from Dos Santos R, Lamas A, Pereigi CJ. L'artériographie des membres de l'aorte et ses branches abdominales. *Bull Soc Nat Chir* 1929; 55:587).

Murray and Best demonstrated that it could prevent thrombosis along suture lines in arteries and venous grafts.

In 1940, Murray summarized the clinical use of heparin, concluding that it was an important agent for prevention of thrombosis during repair of blood vessels, and was valuable in disease states that might promote venous thrombosis (Figure 6.10).

Realization of the great potential value of heparin led to another landmark contribution to vascular surgery: thromboendarterectomy. The early attempts at this procedure by Severeanu in 1880 and Jianu in 1909 were unsuccessful

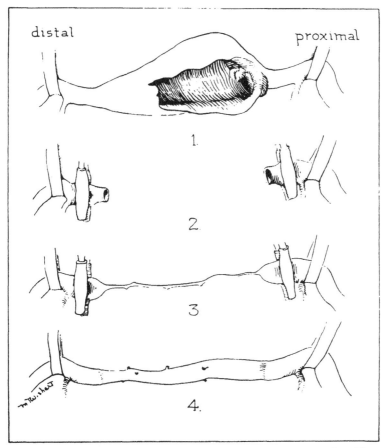

**Figure 6.10** Murray's illustration of venous transplantation with the use of heparin (from Murray G. Heparin in surgical treatment of blood vessels. *Arch Surg* 1940; 40:307).

because of thrombosis. Delbet also attempted thromboendarterectomy in 1906 and, despite his failure, concluded that:

> The easiest operation that can be done to cure arterial obstruction is incision of the artery, extraction of the thrombus and closure of the vessel.

Nevertheless, the procedure was abandoned by surgeons until 1946. Joao Cid Dos Santos (son of Reynaldo), with 3 years of vascular surgical experience with the use of heparin under his belt, conceived the following idea:

> Exactly what I had in mind was to find the plane of cleavage between the old thrombus and the intima, leaving a devastated initial wall to be coated by newly built endothelium while anticoagulation was active.

Dos Santos's first patient was a 66-year-old man with end-stage renal failure and a threatened left lower extremity secondary to an iliac–femoral occlusion. On August 27, 1946, Dos Santos performed the first successful thromboend-arterectomy with a silver ophthalmic spatula and a gallstone scoop. The postoperative angiogram revealed patency of the iliac and femoral arteries (Figure 6.11). The patient died of uremia 2 days later. A second arteriogram performed prior to the autopsy also confirmed arterial patency.

Four months later, Dos Santos saw a 35-year-old woman with ischemia of the right upper extremity caused by occlusion of the subclavian artery. Using the same instruments, a successful thromboendarterectomy was performed again. In 1975, 22 years later, Dos Santos confirmed continued patency of the subclavian artery in his patient.

The significance of Dos Santos's procedures was soon realized by other surgeons such as Bazy in France and Wylie and Freeman in the United States. As a result of their work, thromboendarterectomy became a basic technique in the repertoire of every vascular surgeon.

It is ironic that World War II produced fewer contributions to vascular surgery than World War I. In their review of 2471 acute arterial injuries during the war, DeBakey and Simeone identified only 40 cases of repair with vein grafts, resulting in a 58 percent amputation rate. They concluded that the indications for reconstruction of acute arterial injuries with venous grafts were few.

The story of the venous autograft resumes in Paris. Although initially advocated by Jaeger in 1913, Jean Kunlin revived the technique of bypass grafting in

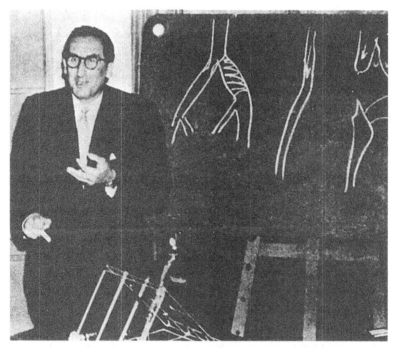

**Figure 6.11** Joao Cid Dos Santos describes his concept of thromboendarterectomy (from Haimovici H. Matas Lecture: The early pioneers in vascular surgery and their legacy. *J Cardiovasc Surg* 1984; 25:275; reprinted by permission).

1948 (see Figure 19.1). His patient was a 54-year-old man on Leriche's service, who, despite a lumbar symphathectomy, a femoral arteriectomy, and a great toe amputation, was still suffering with painful gangrenous ulcers. On June 3, Kunlin harvested a 26-cm length of greater saphenous vein and, because of scarring from prior surgery, performed proximal and distal end-to-end anastomoses between the femoral and popliteal arteries. The concept of an end-to-side anastomosis was a new and important one, as side branches between the anastomoses could now be preserved. The results were dramatic, with healing of the ulcers and resumption of painless walking by the patient. In 1951, Kunlin reported 17 cases of autogenous venous bypasses (see Figure 19.2).

Six months after Kunlin's historic operation, the first successful bypass was performed in the United States by William Holden. His patient was also a young man with lower extremity ischemia of 5 years' duration. The favorable results of Holden's procedure led him to conclude that, despite its appearance as a "radical form of therapy," the alternative of amputation was also radical. He summarized the sentiments of most present-day vascular surgeons with his final comment:

> There are many factors which may jeopardize the success of this procedure, and it is to be hoped that with patience and application they may be eliminated.

In his analysis of 304 vascular injuries during the Korean War, Hughes found 34 cases of autogenous vein graft use, resulting in a limb salvage rate close to 90 percent. Continued evaluation of venous grafts for the treatment of arterial injuries was continued by Rich during the Vietnam War with similar excellent results.

Wider acceptance of the principles of arterial reconstruction continued in civilian practice. In 1951, Fontaine reported 28 cases of venous autografts, with patency of 10 during the follow-up of nearly 1 year.

This procedure was favorably received in the United States, and in 1952 Julian reported 19 cases of bypass grafts with success in 12. Other early series included those of Lord and Stone, who reported 21 autogenous vein grafts in 1957; Dale and DeWeese, who analyzed 31 cases in 1959; and Linton and Darling, who reported on 76 consecutive saphenous vein bypass grafts in 1962.

The efficacy of autogenous venous conduits in the arterial system was established by the end of the 1950s. At that time, several surgeons were contemplating ways to make the procedure faster by leaving the saphenous vein *in situ*. This idea occurred simultaneously in two different centers in 1959. Paul Cartier of Montreal and Karl Hall, while working with Charles Rob in St Mary's Hospital in London, began the first clinical trials of *in situ* vein bypass (Figures 6.12–6.14).

Cartier employed a retrograde valve stripper while Hall, after several unsuccessful cases with a blunt vein stripper introduced antegrade, resorted, upon his return to Norway, to direct excision of the valve cusps. Because this was such a long and tedious procedure, Hall developed his own retrograde valve stripper in 1968. He reported his results in 1978 with the original technique in 252 cases (Figure 6.15). By 1984, Cartier had performed over 850 *in situ* bypasses with a 75 percent 5-year patency rate.

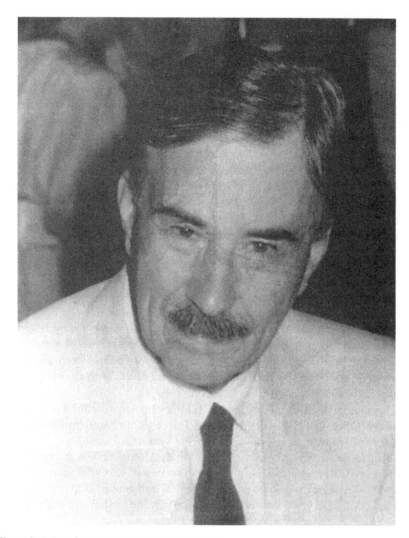

**Figure 6.12**  Paul Cartier (courtesy of Dr. Paul Cartier).

While Cartier and Hall were perfecting their techniques, several discouraging reports of *in situ* vein bypass appeared in the United States. Darling, May, Barner, and others concluded that the *in situ* technique offered no advantage over the reversed technique. The failures with this procedure were primarily due to ineffective or overly traumatic methods of valve disruption. Consequently, the procedure fell into disfavor for nearly a decade until Leather reported excellent results utilizing "a simplified atraumatic method of rendering the valves incompetent" in 1979. Since then, the *in situ* technique has enjoyed a revival and is the preferred method of venous grafting in many centers.

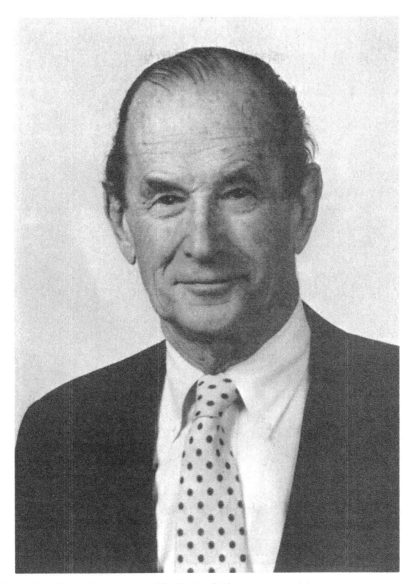

**Figure 6.13** Charles Rob (courtesy of Dr. Charles Rob).

Impressed by the work of Karl Hall, Leather reasoned that a simplified atraumatic method of rendering the saphenous vein valves incompetent could produce better results. He used specially designed microvascular scissors to excise valve leaflets through convenient side branches. Leather reported cumulative patency rates of 91 percent at 12 and 24 months in the initial 89 *in situ* bypasses performed in this manner. He proposed that this technique would allow utiliza-

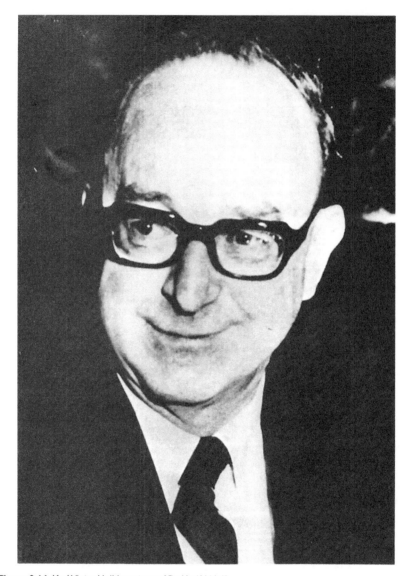

**Figure 6.14** Karl Victor Hall (courtesy of Dr. Karl V. Hall).

tion of veins that were too small for excision and reversal, and that this technique was the superior of the two.

Leather and his coworkers eventually reported long-term results of 2058 *in situ* vein bypasses performed over a 20-year period (1975–1995). The indication for surgery was limb-threatening ischemia in 91 percent of their patients. The cumulative secondary patency rates were 91 percent, 81 percent, and 70 percent after 1, 5, and 10 years respectively. The limb salvage rates at these intervals were

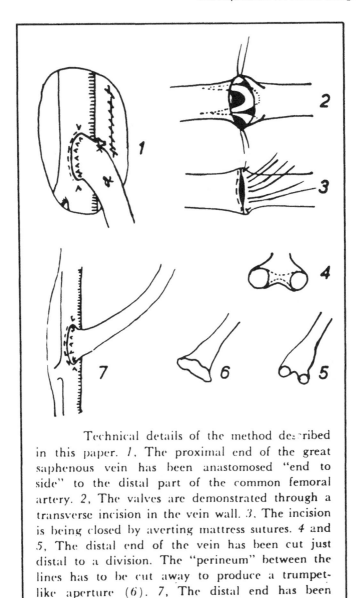

Technical details of the method de:￢ribed in this paper. *1*, The proximal end of the great saphenous vein has been anastomosed "end to side" to the distal part of the common femoral artery. *2*, The valves are demonstrated through a transverse incision in the vein wall. *3*, The incision is being closed by averting mattress sutures. *4* and *5*, The distal end of the vein has been cut just distal to a division. The "perineum" between the lines has to be cut away to produce a trumpet-like aperture (*6*). *7*, The distal end has been anastomosed to the popliteal artery.

**Figure 6.15** Hall's illustration and description of his technique for *in situ* vein bypass (from Hall KV. The great saphenous vein used "in-situ" as an arterial shunt after extirpation of the vein valves. *Surgery* 1962; 51:492).

97 percent, 95 percent, and 90 percent respectively. The authors concluded that the *in situ* saphenous vein was an excellent conduit for limb salvage bypasses.

As surgeons are wont to do, many took sides in the debate over which technique was superior. Stating the case for reversed veins in 1990, Taylor reported the results of a "modern series" of 516 reversed vein bypasses in 387 patients. The indication for surgery was limb salvage in 80 percent of patients, and only 55 percent of limbs possessed adequate ipsilateral saphenous vein. The primary and secondary patency rates for all grafts after 5 years were 75 percent and 81 percent respectively. Taylor preferred the reversed vein technique owing to the excellent patency rates and the value of this procedure in the large number of patients without ipsilateral greater saphenous vein.

One year later, Donaldson provided counterpoise with a report of 440 consecutive *in situ* saphenous vein bypasses in 371 patients, performed during a 7-year period. Limb-threatening ischemia was the indication for surgery in 68 percent of cases. The 5-year secondary patency rate was 83 percent, with an 88 percent limb salvage rate. Based on these results, and the versatility and simplicity of the *in situ* technique, Donaldson concluded that it was the procedure of choice for long infrapopliteal bypasses.

In 1992, Rosenthal described a preliminary multicenter report of endovascular *in situ* saphenous vein bypass. Valvulotomy was accomplished with a long retrograde valvulotome, and steerable nitinol catheters were used to coil embolize saphenous vein branches, all under angioscopic surveillance. The appeal of this procedure was avoiding long leg incisions, reducing wound complications, and reducing hospital stays. Eight years later, he reported favorable cumulative patency, limb salvage, and cost results with this technique after a mean follow-up of 16.6 months.

Voices of reason in this debate took the form of several prospective randomized comparisons of the two techniques, each of which found no significant differences between the two. In one multicenter trial, 125 patients were randomized to receive reversed vein or *in situ* bypasses. After 2.5 years, there was no significant difference in patency rates for the two graft types. The authors of this study noted relative advantages of both techniques and concluded, most importantly: ". . . surgeons performing these operations should be adept at both procedures."

## Bibliography

Barner HB, Judd DR, Kaiser GC, *et al*. Late failure of arterialized in situ saphenous vein. *Arch Surg* 1969; 99:781.

Bazy L, Huguier J, Reboul H, *et al*. Technique des "endarterectomies" pour arterites oblitérantes chroniques des membres inférieurs. *J Chir* (Paris) 1949; 65:196.

Bernheim BM. *Surgery of the Vascular System*. Philadelphia: JB Lippincott Co., 1913.

Bernheim BM. The ideal operation for aneurysm of the extremity. Report of a case. *Bull Johns Hopkins Hosp* 1916; 27:93.

Best CH, Scott C. The purification of heparin. *J Biol Chem* 1933; 102:425.

Brooks B. Injection of sodium iodide. *JAMA* 1924; 82:1016.

Cameron DF. Aqueous solutions of potassium and sodium iodide as opaque medium in roentgenography. *JAMA* 1918; 70:754.

Carrel A. La technique opératoire des anastamoses vasculaires et la transplantation des viscères. *Lyon Med* 1902; 98:859.

Carrel A. The surgery of blood vessels, etc. *Bull Johns Hopkins Hosp* 1907; 190:18.

Carrel A, Guthrie CC. Results of biterminal transplantation of veins. *Am J Med Sci* 1906; 132: 415.

Carrel A, Guthrie CC. Uniterminal and biterminal venous transplantation. *Surg Gynecol Obstet* 1906; 2:266.

Carrel A, Morel A. Anastamose bout à bout de la jugulaire et de la carotide primitive. *Lyon Med* 1902; 99:114.

Dale WA. *Management of Vascular Surgical Problems*. New York: McGraw Hill, 1985.

Dale WA, DeWeese JA, Merle Scott WJ. Autogenous venous shunt grafts. Rationale and report of 31 for atherosclerosis. *Surgery* 1959; 46:145.

Darling RC, Linton RR, Razzuk MA. Saphenous vein bypass grafts for femoropopliteal occlusive disease: A reappraisal. *Surgery* 1967; 31:61.

DeBakey ME, Simeone FA. Battle injuries of the arteries in WW II. An analysis of 2471 cases. *Ann Surg* 1946; 123:534.

Delbet P. *Chirurgie artérielle et veineuse. Les modernes acquisitions*. Paris: JB Bailliere et Fils, 1906.

Donaldson MC, Whittemore AD, Mannick JA. Femoral-distal bypass with in situ greater saphenous vein. Long-term results using the Mills valvulotome. *Ann Surg* 1991; 213:457.

Donaldson MC, Whittemore AD, Mannick JA. Further experience with an all-autogenous tissue policy for infrainguinal reconstruction. *J Vasc Surg* 1993; 18:41.

Dos Santos JC. Leriche memorial lecture. From embolectomy to endarterectomy or the fall of myth. *J Cardiovasc Surg* 1976; 17:113.

Dos Santos R, Lamas A, Pereirgi CJ. L'artériographie des membres de l'aorte et ses branches abdominales. *Bull Soc Nat Chir* 1929; 55:587.

Exner A. Einige tierversuche ueber vereinigung und transplantation von blutgefaessen. *Wien Klin Wschr* 1903; 16:273.

Fogle MA, Whittemore AD, Couch NP, et al. A comparison of in situ and reversed saphenous vein grafts for infrainguinal reconstruction. *J Vasc Surg* 1987; 5:46.

Fontaine R, Buck P, Riveaux R, et al. Treatment of arterial occlusion, comparative value of thrombectomy, thromboendarterectomy, arteriovenous shunt and vascular grafts (fresh venous autografts). *Lyon Chir* 1951; 46:73.

Freeman NE, Gilfillan RS. Regional heparinization after thromboendarterectomy in the treatment of obliterative arterial disease: Preliminary report based on 12 cases. *Surgery* 1952; 31:115.

Gluck T. Die moderne chirurgie des circulationapparats. *Berl Klin* 1898; 70:1.

Goyanes J. Nuevos trabajos de cirugia vascular. Substitucion plastica de las arterias por las venas, o arterioplastia venosa, applicada, como nuevo metodo, al tratamiento de los aneurismas. *El Siglo Med* 1906; Sept:346, 561.

Hall KV. The great saphenous vein used "in-situ" as an arterial shunt after extirpation of the vein valves. *Surgery* 1962; 51:492.

Hall KV. The saphenous vein used "in-situ" as an arterial bupass. *Am J Surg* 1978; 136:123.

Harris PL, How TV, Jones DR. Prospectively randomized clinical trial to compare in situ and reversed saphenous vein grafts for femoropopliteal bypass. *Br J Surg* 1987; 74:252.

Harrison LH Jr. Historical aspects in the development of venous autografts. *Ann Surg* 1976; 183:101.

Haschek E, Lindenthal OT. Ein beitrag zur praktischen verwerthung der photographie nach Roentgen. *Wien Klin Wochenschr* 1896; 9:63.

Hoepfner E. Ueber gefaessnaht, gefaesstransplantation und replantation von amputierten extremitaeten. *Arch Klin Chir* 1903; 70:417.

Holden WD. Reconstruction of the femoral artery for arteriosclerotic thrombosis. *Surgery* 1950; 27:417.

Howell WH. Two new factors in blood coagulation – heparin and proantithrombin. *Am J Physiol* 1918; 47:328.

Hughes CW. Arterial repair during the Korean War. *Ann Surg* 1958; 147:555.

Jaeger E. *Die Chirurgie der Blutgefaesse und des Herzens*. Berlin: A Hirsrchwald, 1913.

Jaeger E. Zur technik der blutgefaessnaht. *Beitr Klin Chir* 1915; 97:553.

Jianu I. Trombectomia arteriala pentru un caz de gangrena uscata a piciorului. *Soc Chir* (Bucarest) 1912; 27:11.

Julian OC, Dye WS, Olwin JH. Direct surgery of arteriosclerosis. *Ann Surg* 1952; 136:459.

Kunlin J. Le traitement de l'artérite obliterante par la greffe veineuse. *Arch Mal Coeur* 1949; 42:371.

Kunlin J. Le traitement de l'ischemie artéritique par la greffe veineuse longue. *Rev Chir* 1951; 70:206.

Leather RP, Powers SR Jr., Karmody AM. The reappraisal of the in situ saphenous vein arterial bypass: Its use in limb salvage. *Surgery* 1979; 86:453.

Lexer E. Die ideale operation des arteriellen und des arteriellvenoesen aneurysma. *Arch Klin Chir* 1907; 83:459.

Lexer E. Zwanzig jahre transplantationsforschung in der chirurgie. *Arch Klin Chir* 1925; 138:251.

Linton RR, Darling RC. Autogenous saphenous vein bypass grafts in femoropopliteal obliterative arterial disease. *Surgery* 1962; 51:62.

Lord JW, Stone DW. The use of autologous venous grafts in the peripheral arterial system. *Arch Surg* 1957; 74:71.

MacLean J. The thromboplastic action of cephalin. *Am J Physiol* 1916; 41:250.

May AG, DeWeese JA, Rob CG. Arteialized in situ saphenous vein. *Arch Surg* 1965; 91:743.

Moniz E. L'éncephalographie artérielle son importance dans la localisation des tumeurs cérébrales. *Rev Neurol* 1927; 2:72.

Moody AP, Edwards PR, Harris PL. In situ versus reversed femoropopliteal vein grafts: long-term follow-up of a prospective, randomized trial. *Br J Surg* 1992; 79:750.

Murray G. Heparin in surgical treatment of blood vessels. *Arch Surg* 1940; 40:307.

Payr E. Weitere mittheilungen ueber verwendung des magnesiums bei der naht der blutgefaesse. *Arch Klin Chir* 1901; 64:726.

Porter JM. In situ versus reversed vein graft: Is one superior. *J Vasc Surg* 1987; 5:779.

Pringle H. Two cases of vein grafting for the maintenance of direct arterial circulation. *Lancet* 1913; 1:1795.

Rich NM. Vascular trauma in Vietnam. *J Cardiovasc Surg* 1970; 11:368.

Roentgen WK. Ueber sine neue art von Strahlen (trans). *Nature* 1896; 53:274.

Rosenthal D, Herring MB, O'Donovan TG, *et al*. Endovascular infrainguinal in situ saphenous vein bypass: A multicenter preliminary report. *J Vasc Surg* 1992; 16:453.

Rosenthal D, Arous EJ, Friedman SG, *et al*. Endovascular-assisted versus conventional in situ saphenous vein bypass grafting: Cumulative patency, limb salvage, and cost results in a 39-month multicenter study. *J Vasc Surg* 2000; 31:60.

Shah DM, Darlin, RC III, Chang BB, *et al*. Long-term results of in situ vein bypass. Analysis of 2058 cases. *Ann Surg* 1995; 222:438.

Sicard A, Forestier J. L'huile iodée en clinique; applications thérapeutiques et diagnostiques. *Bull Mem Hosp Paris* 1923; 47:309.

Stich R, Makkas M, Dowman CE. Beitrage zur gefaesschirurgie; cirkulaere arteriennaht und gefaesstransplantationen. *Beitr Klin Chir* 1907; 53:113.

Taylor LM Jr., Edwards JM, Phinney ES, *et al.* Reversed vein bypass to infrapopliteal arteries. Modern results are superior to or equivalent to in situ bypass for patency and for vein utilization. *Ann Surg* 1987; 205:90.

Taylor LM Jr., Edwards JM, Porter JM. Present status of reversed vein bypass grafting: Five year results of a modern series. *J Vasc Surg* 1990; 11:193.

Warthmuller H. Ueber die bisherigen erfolge der gefaesstransplantation am menschen. *Dis G Neuenbann Jena* 1917.

Weglowski R. Ueber die gefaesstransplantation. *Zentr Chir* 1925; 52:441.

Wengerter KR, Veith FJ, Gupta SK, *et al.* Prospective randomized multicenter comparison of in situ and reversed vein infrapopliteal bypasses. *J Vasc Surg* 1991; 13:189.

Wylie EJ. Thromboendarterectomy for arteriosclerotic thrombosis of major arteries. *Surgery* 1952; 32:275.

# CHAPTER 7

# Evolution of aortic surgery

*Life shrinks or expands in proportion to one's courage.*

(*Anaïs Nin*)

The original operations on the aorta were for the treatment of aneurysms. Arterial reconstruction was an unknown concept until the 20th century, and ligation of the aorta appeared to be the best treatment for these lesions. The first case has already been described. It took place in 1817, when Astley Cooper ligated the aortic bifurcation in a 38-year-old man for a ruptured left external iliac aneurysm. Cooper performed the surgery while the patient was still in his hospital bed. Although the first postoperative day passed smoothly, the patient died on the second day following surgery.

The second case of aortic ligation was also performed for an aneurysm of the left external iliac artery. It was undertaken in 1829, when J.H. James ligated the aortic bifurcation in a 44-year-old man. His patient succumbed to shock 4 hours after the surgery.

Prior to the turn of the 20th century, 10 additional cases of aortic ligation were recorded. Most of these were for syphilitic aneurysms of the iliac arteries in young men ranging in age from 28 to 52 years. In eight cases, the aortic bifurcation was ligated, and in another case ligation was performed just below the renal arteries. Most of these cases resulted in death from hemorrhagic shock within hours. The longest survivor was a patient of Keen, who underwent aortic ligation at the diaphragm for a ruptured abdominal aortic aneurysm in 1899. The surgery was successful and the patient survived 48 days, at which time the aortic ligature eroded into the vessel.

The first aortic ligation in the 20th century, by Tillaux, emphasized the paucity of progress since Cooper's original procedure. Tillaux ligated the aortic bifurcation for a ruptured iliac aneurysm just as Cooper had done. His patient also died within 2 days.

R.T. Morris introduced the first alteration of Cooper's operation in 1901, when he ligated the aortic bifurcation with a soft rubber catheter, hoping to prevent erosion of the ligature into the vessel. His patient, a 24-year-old woman, died 53 hours after the surgery, from ischemic bowel.

Between 1906 and 1911, William Halstead performed four aortic ligations with aluminum bands, also in an attempt to prevent erosion (Figure 7.1). In one case he performed partial ligation of the aorta, and his patient survived for 47 days. Sepsis resulting from an infected band was the cause of death. In one of Halstead's cases, the aneurysm ruptured 18 days after the surgery and in another the band cut through the aorta after 6 weeks.

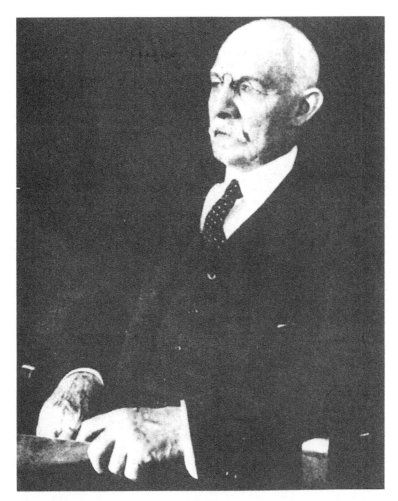

**Figure 7.1** William Halstead (from Rutkow IM. The letters of William Halstead and Erwin Payr. *Surg Gynecol Obstet* 1985; 161:75; reprinted by permission).

The thoracic aorta was not spared from attempts at ligation for aneurysm, and it was Tuffier who attempted the first of these in 1902 (Figure 7.2). His operation was as daring as Cooper's 85 years earlier. Tuffier's patient had a saccular aneurysm of the ascending aorta. Tuffier doubly ligated the neck of the aneurysm with catgut suture and then attempted to dissect it free of surrounding structures to excise it. He abandoned this effort because of the size of the aneurysm and his patient died of sudden hemorrhage on the 13th postoperative day owing to necrosis of the sac. Three subsequent thoracic aortic ligations by Tuffier were also unsuccessful.

In 1914, Kummell reported his attempt to treat a ruptured thoracic aneurysm by oversewing the defect. Although the procedure took only 1 hour, the 52-year-old patient soon "died of exhaustion."

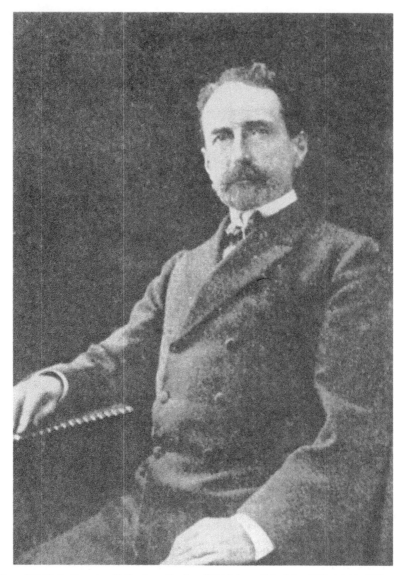

**Figure 7.2** Marin-Theodore Tuffier (from Garrison FH. *History of Medicine*. Philadelphia: WB Saunders Co., 1929).

George Vaughan reported the first long-term success following partial aortic occlusion for an aneurysm in 1921. His patient survived for 2 years and 1 month following aortic ligation with cotton tape.

As previously noted, Rudolph Matas carried out the first successful ligation of the aorta in April 1923, more than a century after Astley Cooper's original attempt (Figure 7.3). Matas's patient was a 28-year-old female plantation worker

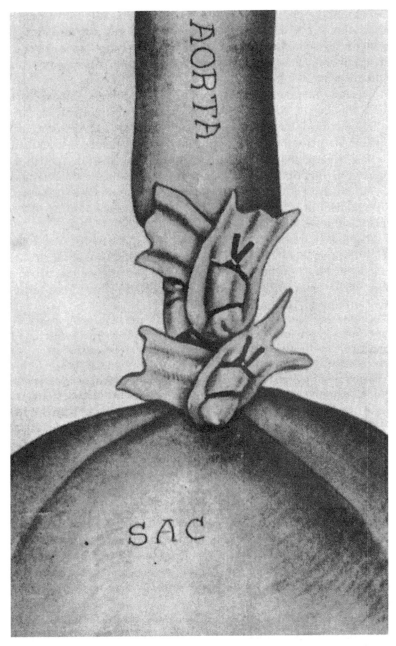

**Figure 7.3** Matas's successful ligation of the abdominal aorta (from Matas R. Aneurysm of the abdominal aorta at its bifurcation into the common iliac arteries. A pictorial supplement illustrating the history of Corrinne D, previously reported as the first recorded instance of cure of an aneurysm of the abdominal aorta by ligation. *Ann Surg* 1940; 112:909).

with a ruptured syphilitic aneurysm of the aortic bifurcation and common iliac arteries. Although Matas had previously experimented with introducing wire into aneurysms to induce thrombosis, he used two cotton tapes to completely ligate the abdominal aorta just above the sac. Matas's patient survived for 17 months, then died of tuberculosis.

At this time, René Leriche (see Figure 18.1) was adding significant contributions to the already formidable list compiled by his predecessors Mathieu Jaboulay and Alexis Carrel. Leriche originally popularized sympathectomy for the treatment of arterial occlusive disease. He also attempted several autogenous vein bypasses of occluded iliac segments unsuccessfully. Leriche is best known for his description of "obliteration of the terminal abdominal aorta" in 1923. He anticipated the present treatment of this lesion when he wrote: "The ideal treatment of arterial thrombosis is the replacement of the obliterated segment with a vascular graft."

Little progress in aortic surgery occurred during the two decades following Matas's historic operation. Scattered reports of successful aortic ligation appeared in the literature, but surgeons remained hesitant to undertake this procedure. Bigger summarized the prevailing attitude when he addressed the American Surgical Association in 1940:

> Judging from the literature, only a small number of surgeons have felt that direct surgical attack upon aneurysms of the abdominal aorta was justifiable, and it must be admitted that the results obtained by surgical intervention have been discouraging.

That many surgeons still feared direct surgical treatment of aortic aneurysms was demonstrated by the resurrection of techniques to introduce foreign material into them to promote thrombosis. The first attempt was by Alfred Velpeau in 1831, with three pairs of sewing needles being introduced (Figure 7.4). Moore used 26 yards of iron wire in 1865, and Corradi modified this technique in 1879 by passing an electric current through the wire. Blakemore and King experimented with this method in 1938. Cellophane wrapping was also investigated by Pearse in 1940, and by Harrison 3 years later. Many other surgeons examined these therapeutic alternatives.

Enthusiasm for aortic surgery was renewed in 1944 when Alexander and Byron reported the first successful excision of an aortic aneurysm with proximal and distal ligation (Figure 7.5). Their patient was a 19-year-old college student with an 18-cm thoracic aneurysm. Except for persistent headaches and hypertension, the patient made a good recovery and was discharged on the 37th postoperative day.

In the case of Alexander's patient, the aneurysm was due to coarctation of the aorta. Surgical attempts at treating this lesion during the 1940s played an important role in the development of aortic surgery and heralded operations upon the aorta for lesions other than aneurysms. In 1944, Blalock and Park hypothesized that the left subclavian artery could be used to bypass a coarctation, but it was Clarence Crafoord of Sweden who performed the first successful correction of this condition

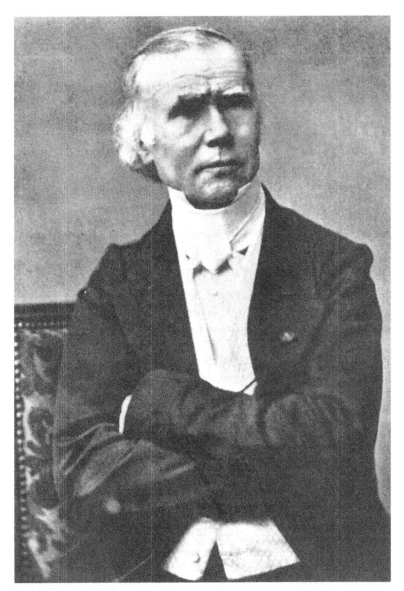

**Figure 7.4** Alfred Armand Louis Marie Velpeau (from Major RA. *A History of Medicine.* Springfield, IL: Charles C Thomas, 1954).

(Figure 7.6). On October 19 and 31, 1944, Crafoord resected coarctations in a 12-year-old schoolboy and a 27-year-old farmer respectively. In each case the aorta was repaired by end-to-end anastomosis using the triangulation technique of Carrel. Both patients made excellent recoveries following brief respiratory tract infections.

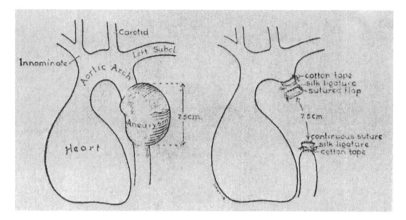

**Figure 7.5** The operation of Alexander and Byron (from Alexander J, Byron FX. Aortectomy for thoracic aneurysm. *JAMA* 1944; 126:1139).

In June 1945, Robert Gross repeated this procedure in the United States (Figure 7.7). An end-to-end aortic anastomosis was also performed by Shumacker during the first successful aortic aneurysm resection with restoration of arterial continuity in 1947 (Figure 7.8). Shumacker's patient was an 8-year-old boy with a thoracic aortic coarctation and a 4-cm aneurysm.

During the next few years, surgical correction of aortic coarctation was performed in many centers throughout the world, with excellent results. This was a critical period in aortic surgery as surgeons began to realize their ability to clamp and suture the aorta without disrupting its integrity.

The next contribution to aortic surgery was made through efforts to reconstruct the aorta when end-to-end anastomosis was not possible. Surgical researchers had endeavored to find ways to successfully bridge large gaps in arteries since the work of Abbe in 1894. Only after many years of experimentation was it accepted that the use of rigid arterial prostheses was not feasible.

The original experiments with implantation of preserved blood vessels were performed by Carrel and Guthrie in Chicago. They replaced cat abdominal aortas with canine veins and arteries that had been harvested several weeks earlier and preserved near the freezing point of water in a salt solution. One of their heterografts remained patent for 77 days. Carrel continued this work following his move to Rockefeller University.

The first successful operations for aortic coarctation brought about a renewed interest in arterial homografts. Blakemore and Lord, Huffnagel, and Pierce and Gross all studied the possibility of replacing human arteries with those previously harvested and stored by a variety of methods.

In 1948, Gross reported the preliminary use of preserved arterial grafts in humans with cyanotic heart disease and coarctation. That same year Swan used

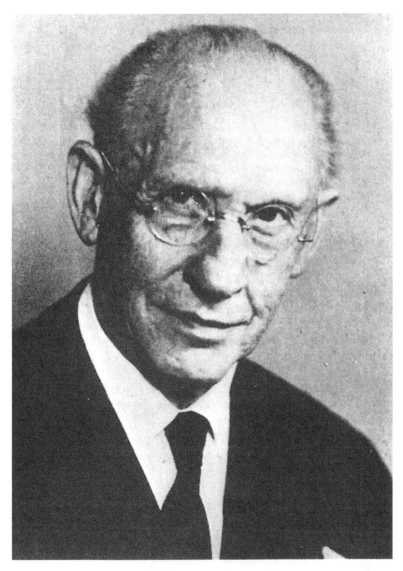

**Figure 7.6** Clarence Crafoord (from Bjork VO. Clarence Crafoord (1900–1984) the leading European thoracic surgeon died. *J Cardiovasc Surg* 1984; 25:473; reprinted by permission from Appleton-Century-Crofts).

an arterial homograft following resection of a thoracic aneurysm in a 16-year-old boy. These initial successful treatments of aneurysms and coarctations with homografts quickly led to their use in the treatment of aorto-iliac occlusive disease.

The line of great French vascular surgeons was extended by Jacques

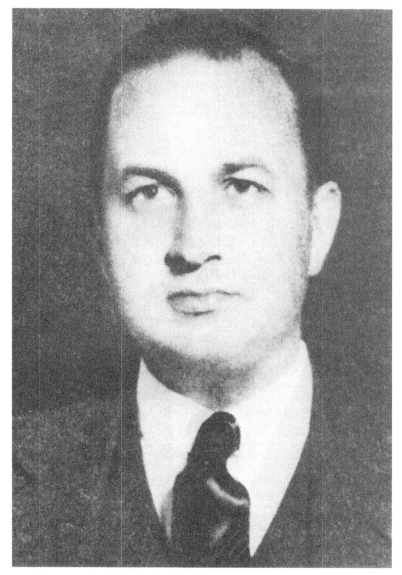

**Figure 7.7** Robert Gross (from Callow AD. Historical development of vascular grafts. In: Sawyer PN, Kaplitt MJ, eds. *Vascular Grafts*. New York: Appleton-Century-Crofts, 1978).

Oudot when he replaced a thrombosed aortic bifurcation with an arterial homograft in November 1950. Following persistent ischemia of the right lower extremity, he placed a second homograft from the left to the right external iliac artery. The patient made an excellent recovery and over the next 2 years Oudot performed four more aortic bifurcation resections with homograft

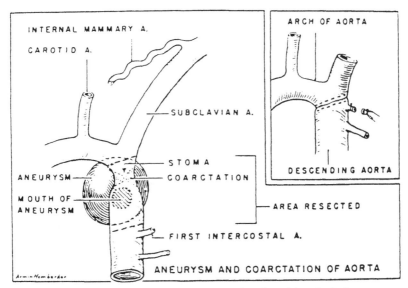

INTERNAL MAMMARY A.

CAROTID A.

SUBCLAVIAN A.

ARCH OF AORTA

DESCENDING AORTA

STOMA

ANEURYSM

COARCTATION

MOUTH OF
ANEURYSM

AREA RESECTED

FIRST INTERCOSTAL A.

ANEURYSM AND COARCTATION OF AORTA

**Figure 7.8** Shumacker's aneurysm resection with restoration of arterial continuity (from Shumacker HB Jr. Coarctation and aneurysm of the aorta. Report of a case treated by excision and end-to-end suture of aorta. *Ann Surg* 1948; 127:655).

replacement (Figure 7.9). The 27-year-old prophecy of René Leriche had been fulfilled.

In March 1951, Charles Dubost, also of France, resected an abdominal aortic aneurysm in a 50-year-old man and restored arterial continuity with a thoracic aortic homograft harvested from a young girl 3 weeks previously (see Figures 20.1 and 20.2). These techniques were soon adopted in the United States by Julian, DeBakey, and Szilagyi.

One month prior to Dubost's operation, Freeman excised an abdominal aortic aneurysm in a 61-year-old woman, and restored arterial continuity with one of her common iliac veins. The patient died 6 hours after surgery. Freeman attempted this procedure in three more patients, with good results in one.

The enthusiasm for homografts during the decade from 1945 to 1955 was similar to the enthusiasm for rigid arterial prostheses 50 years earlier. Both methods were quickly embraced by surgeons throughout the world as a sure way to bridge arterial defects. Almost as quickly, however, interest in both techniques waned. The popularity of rigid prostheses lasted for two decades until it became clear that they all eventually thrombosed. The use of homografts was even more short-lived owing to degenerative changes resulting in poor long-term patency rates, and the difficulties associated with harvesting and preserving them. The brief homograft period was an important one, however, as it enabled surgeons to become skillful in performing operations upon the aorta. It also led directly to attempts to use synthetic fabrics as vascular conduits, thereby ushering in the present era of reconstructive arterial surgery.

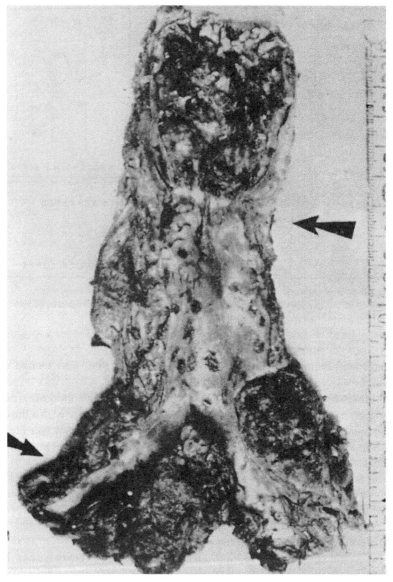

**Figure 7.9** Resected aortic bifurcation from Oudot's second case of homograft replacement for aortic occlusion (from Oudot J, Beaconsfield P. Thrombosis of the aortic bifurcation treated by resection and homograft replacement. Report of five cases. *Arch Surg* 1953; 66:365).

During the ensuing decades, vascular surgeons happily set about reconstructing thousands of aortas with these new prostheses. An abundance of experience was garnered, validating the efficacy and durability of aortic replacement with fabric tubes.

Large series of patients began appearing in the literature in the 1970s. In 1978, Brewster compared aortic endarterectomy with grafting in 582 patients over a 15-year period. He concluded that aortic grafts could be performed with low mortality and superior long-term results.

In 1981, Crawford reported a 25-year experience with aortoiliac reconstruction in 1004 patients. He too noted a low mortality rate, particularly in the last 15 years of the study, and a high rate of limb salvage and symptom relief.

In 1986, Szilagyi weighed in with his 30-year experience with the treatment of aortoiliac disease. He reported the outcome of 1748 procedures in 1647 patients. Complete follow-up was obtained in 94 percent of his patients. Patency rates for aortofemoral bypasses were 77 percent after 5 and 10 years, 73 percent after 15 years, and 68 percent after 20 years.

One year later, Burke suggested that polytetrafluoroethylene (PTFE) bifurcation grafts were superior to Dacron grafts in patients with small aortas (14 mm or less).

The results of these and other similar studies validated aortoiliac reconstruction with fabric prostheses as the most durable form of arterial reconstruction in the vascular surgery repertoire.

In the 1990s, surgeons turned their attention toward less invasive techniques for aortic reconstruction. The outstanding example of this was Parodi's landmark description, in 1991, of transfemoral intraluminal graft implantation for abdominal aortic aneurysms.

In 1996, Chen reported the results of laparoscopically assisted abdominal aortic aneurysm repair in 10 patients. She suggested that early removal of nasogastric tubes, shorter stays in intensive care, and earlier discharge were potential advantages. Several other studies of this technique have been reported, but it has not gained popularity.

In a similar vein, Matsumoto recently described the use of a minilaparotomy to repair abdominal aortic aneurysms. He too suggested that faster recovery and reduced lengths of stay could be achieved with this technique.

## Bibliography

Abbott W, Osler A. Clinical experiences with the application of polythene cellophane upon aneurysms of the thoracic vessels. *J Thorac Surg* 1949; 18:435.

Alexander J, Byron FX. Aortectomy for thoracic aneurysm. *JAMA* 1944; 126:1139.

Allen R. Presidential address: The evolution of pediatric surgery. *J Ped Surg* 1980; 15:711.

Bigger IA. The surgical treatment of aneurysm of the abdominal aorta. Review of the literature and report of two cases, one apparently successful. *Ann Surg* 1940; 112:879.

Bing RJ, Handelsman JC, Campbell JA, *et al*. The surgical treatment and the physiopathology of coarctation of the aorta. *Ann Surg* 1948; 128:803.

Bjork VO. Clarence Crafoord (1900–1984) the leading European thoracic surgeon died. *J Cardiovasc Surg* 1984; 25:473.

Blakemore A. Progressive constrictive occlusion of the abdomimal aorta with wiring and electrothermic coagulation. A one-stage operation for arteriosclerotic aneurysms of the abdominal aorta. *Ann Surg* 1951; 133:447.

Blakemore A, King BG. Electrothermic coagulation of aortic aneurysms. *JAMA* 1938; 111:1821.

Blakemore A, Lord J. A non-suture method of blood vessel anastomosis. *Ann Surg* 1945;121:435.

Brewster DC, Darling C. Optimal methods of aortoiliac reconstruction. *Surgery* 1978; 84:739.

Brooks B. Ligation of the aorta. A clinical and experimental study. *JAMA* 1926; 87:722.

Burke PM Jr., Herrmann JB, Cutler BS. Optimal grafting methods for the small abdominal aorta. *J Cardiovasc Surg* 1987; 28:420.

Carrel A. Heterotransplantation of blood vessels preserved in cold storage. *J Exp Med* 1907; 9:226.

Carrel A. The preservation of tissues and its application in surgery. *JAMA* 1912; 59:523.

Carrel A. Ultimate results of aortic transplantation. *J Exp Med* 1912; 15:389.

Castronuovo JJ Jr., James KV, Resnikoff M, *et al*. Laparoscopic-assisted abdominal aortic aneurysmectomy. *J Vasc Surg* 2000; 32:224.

Cerveira JJ, Halpern VJ, Faust G, Cohen JR. Minimal incision abdominal aortic aneurysm repair. *J Vasc Surg* 1999; 30:977–84.

Chen MH, D'Angelo AJ, Murphy EA, *et al*. Laparoscopically assisted abdominal aortic aneurysm repair. A report of 10 cases. *Surg Endosc* 1996; 10:1136.

Cooley DA, DeBakey ME. Surgical considerations of intrathoracic aneurysms of the aorta and great vessels. *Ann Surg* 1952; 135:660.

Crafoord C, Nylin G. Congenital coarctation of the aorta and its surgical treatment. *J Thorac Surg* 1945; 14:347.

Crawford ES, Bomberger RA, Glaeser DH, *et al*. Aortoiliac occlusive disease: Factors influencing survival and function following reconstructive operation over a twenty-five-year period. *Surgery* 1981; 90:1055.

DeBakey ME, Cooley DA. Successful resection of aneurysm of thoracic aorta and replacement by graft. *JAMA* 1953; 152:673.

DeBakey ME, Creech O Jr., Cooley DA. Occlusive disease of the aorta and its treatment by resection and homograft replacement. *Ann Surg* 1954; 140:290.

DeTakats G, DeOliveira R. The surgical treatment of aneurysm of the abdominal aorta. *Surgery* 1947; 21:4.

Deterling RA Jr., Coleman C Jr., Parshley MS. Experimental studies of the frozen homologous aortic graft. *Surgery* 1951; 29:419.

Dubost C. First successful resection of an aneurysm of an abdominal aorta with restoration of the continuity by a human arterial graft. *World J Surg* 1982; 6:256.

Dubost C, Allary M, Oeconomos N. Resection of an aneurysm of the abdominal aorta: Reestablishment of the continuity by a preserved human arterial graft, with results after five months. *Arch Surg* 1952; 64:405.

Elkin DC. Aneurysm of the abdominal aorta. Treatment by ligation. *Ann Surg* 1940; 112:895.

Elkin DC, Cooper FW Jr. Surgical treatment of insidious thrombosis of the aorta. *Ann Surg* 1949; 130:417.

Freeman NE, Leeds FH. Vein inlay graft in the treatment of aneurysms and thrombosis of the abdominal aorta. *Angiology* 1951; 2:79.

Garrison FH. *History of Medicine*. Philadelphia: WB Saunders Co., 1929.

Gross RE. Treatment of certain aortic coarctations by homologous grafts. A report of nineteen cases. *Ann Surg* 1951; 134:753.

Gross RE, Hurwitt ES, Bill AH Jr., *et al*. Preliminary observations on the use of human arterial grafts in the treatment of certain cardiovascular defects. *N Engl J Med* 1948; 239: 578.

Gross RE, Bill AH Jr., Pierce EC II. Methods for preservation and transplantation of arterial grafts. Observations on arterial grafts in dogs. Report of transplantation of preserved arterial grafts in 9 human cases. *Surg Gynecol Obstet* 1949; 88:689.

Guthrie CC. End results of arterial restitution with devitalized tissue. *JAMA* 1919; 73:186.

Halsted WS. *Surgical Papers, I*. Baltimore: Johns Hopkins Press, 1924.

Hamann CA. Ligation of the abdominal aorta: Ligation of the first portion of the left subclavian. *Ann Surg* 1918; 268:217.

Harrison PW, Chandy J. A subclavian aneurysm cured by cellophane fibrosis. *Ann Surg* 1943; 118:478.

Hufnagel CE. Preserved homologous arterial transplants. *Bull Am Coll Surg*, Sept 11, 1947.

Julian OC, Dye WS, Olwin JH, *et al*. Direct surgery of arteriosclerosis. *Ann Surg* 1952; 136:459.

Kline RG, D'Angelo AJ, Chen MH, *et al*. Laparoscopically assisted abdominal aortic aneurysm repair: the first 20 cases. *J Vasc Surg* 1998; 27:81.

Kümmell H. Operative treatment of aneurysm of the aorta. *Surg Gynecol Obstet* 1914; 19:163.

Lam CR, Aram HH. Resection of the descending thoracic aorta for aneurysm. A report of the use of a homograft in a case and an experimental study. *Ann Surg* 1951; 134:743.

Leriche R. Des oblitérielles hautes (oblitération de la terminaison de l'aorte) comme cause des insuffisances circulatoires des membres inférieure. *Bull Mem Soc Chir*, Décembre, 1923.

Leriche R, Morel A. The syndrome of thrombotic obliteration of the aortic bifurcation. *Ann Surg* 1948; 127:193.

Levin I, Larkin JH. Transplantation of devitalized arterial segments. *Proc Soc Exp Biol Med* 1907; 5:109.

Matas R. Surgery of the vascular system. In Keen WW, ed. *Surgery, its Principles and Practice*. Philadelphia: WB Saunders Co, 1914.

Matas R. Aneurysm of the abdominal aorta at its bifurcation into the common iliac arteries. A pictorial supplement illustrating the history of Corrinne D, previously reported as the first recorded instance of cure of an aneurysm of the abdominal aorta by ligation. *Ann Surg* 1940; 112:909.

Matsumoto M, Hata T, Tsushima Y, *et al*. The treatment of abdominal aortic aneurysm by minimally invasive vascular surgery (MIVS). *Jpn J Vasc Surg* 2000; 9:389.

Matsumoto M, Hata T, Tsushima Y, *et al*. Minimally invasive vascular surgery for repair of infrarenal abdominal aortic aneurysm with iliac involvement. *J Vasc Surg* 2002; 35: 654.

Middleman IC, Drey NW. Cellophane wrapping of an abdominal aortic aneurysm. *Surg* 1951; 29:890.

Moore CH, Murchison C. On a method of procuring the consolidation of fibrin in certain incurable aneurysms. With the report of a case in which an aneurysm of the ascending aorta was treated by the insertion of wire. *Med Chir Trans* 1864; 47:129.

Oudot J. La greffe vasculaire dans les thromboses du carrefour aortique. *Presse Med* 1951; 59:234.

Oudot J, Beaconsfield P. Thrombosis of the aortic bifurcation treated by resection and homograft replacement. Report of five cases. *Arch Surg* 1953; 66:365.

Parodi JC, Elliott JP Jr., Smith RF, *et al*. A thirty-year survey of the reconstructive surgical treatment of aortoiliac disease. *J Vasc Surg* 1986; 3:21.

Parodi JC, Palmaz JC, Barone HD. Transfemoral intraluminal graft implantation for abdominal aortic aneurysms. *Ann Vasc Surg* 1991; 5:491.

Pearse HE. Experimental studies on the gradual occlusion of large arteries. *Ann Surg* 1940; 112:923.

Peirce EC II, Gross RE, Bill AH Jr. Tissue-culture evaluation of the viability of blood vessels stored by refrigeration. *Ann Surg* 1949; 129:333.

Poppe JK. Cellophane treatment of syphilitic aneurysms with report of results in six cases. *Am Heart J* 1948; 36:252.

Poppe JK, DeOliveira HR. Treatment of syphilitic aneurysms by cellophane wrapping. *J Thorac Surg* 1946; 15:186.

Reid MR. Aneurysms in the Johns Hopkins Hospital. All cases treated in the surgical service from the opening of the hospital to January 1922. *Arch Surg* 1926; 12:1.

Shumacker HB Jr. Coarctation and aneurysm of the aorta. Report of a case treated by excision and end-to-end suture of aorta. *Ann Surg* 1948; 127:655.

Swan H, Maaske C, Johnson M, *et al.* Arterial homografts. II. Resection of thoracic aortic aneurysms using a stored human arterial transplant. *Arch Surg* 1950; 61:732.

Szilagyi DE. Ten years' experience with aorto-iliac and femoropopliteal arterial reconstruction. *J Cardiovasc Surg* 1964; 5:502.

Tuffier T. Intervention chirurgicale directe pour un anevrysme de la crosse de l'aorte ligature du sac. *Press Med* 1902; 23:267.

Turnipseed WD. A less-invasive minilaparotomy technique for repair of aortic aneurysm and occlusive disease. *J Vasc Surg* 2001; 33:431.

Turnipseed WD, Hoch JR, Acher CW, Carr SC. Less invasive aortic surgery: the minilaparotomy technique. *Surgery* 2000; 128:751.

Vaughan GT. Ligation (partial occlusion) of the abdominal aorta for aneurysm. Report of a recent case with a resume of previous cases. *Ann Surg* 1921; 74:308.

Vaughan GT. Ligation of the aorta. Necropsy two years and one month after operation. *Ann Surg* 1922; 76:519.

Velpeau AA. Mémoire sur la figure de l'acupuncture des artères dans le traitement des anevrismes. *Gaz Med (Paris)* 1831; 2:1.

# CHAPTER 8

# Operation on the carotid artery

*... two branches which they call carotids or soporales, the sleepy arteries, because they being obstructed or any way stopt we presently fall asleep ...*

(Ambroise Paré)

The Ancient Greeks first demonstrated some knowledge of the importance of the carotid arteries, as evidenced by the etymology of "carotid," derived from the Greek *karoo*, which meant "to stupefy." Compression of these vessels was thought to plunge one into deep sleep or to cause behavioral changes.

Thomas Willis first recognized the significance of a totally occluded carotid artery in 1684 (Figure 8.1). He encountered this condition in postmortem examinations and eventually described the network that would later bear his name, whereby the four arteries of the brain communicate. Willis discussed the function of the circle in his classic work, *Cerebri Anatome:*

> But there is another reason far greater than this of these manifold ingraftings of the Vessels, to wit, that there may be a manifold way, and that more certain, for the blood about to go into divers Regions of the Brain, laid open for each; so that if by chance one or two should be stopt, there might easily be found another passage instead of them: as for example, if the Carotid of one side might provide for either Province .... Further, if both the Carotids should be stopt, the offices of each might be supplied through the vertebrals.

The first surgery upon the carotid artery was ligation for hemorrhage; it was performed by Hebenstreit in 1793.

In 1798, John Abernethy was asked to see a patient who was bleeding profusely from a puncture wound in the left neck delivered by a bull's horn (Figure 8.2). He arrested the hemorrhage by compression and then ligated the carotid artery.

Astley Cooper performed the first carotid artery ligation for aneurysm in 1805 on a 44-year-old woman with a large pulsatile mass of the right neck. As noted earlier, his patient initially did well following surgery but died of an infection on the 16th postoperative day. Three years later, Cooper repeated this procedure in a 50-year-old man with a left carotid artery aneurysm. The patient survived until 1821, when he succumbed to a left-sided cerebral hemorrhage.

Benjamin Travers performed common carotid artery ligation in 1809 for a carotid–cavernous sinus fistula (Figure 8.3). It appears that surgeons of the 19th century were quite willing to ligate the carotid for hemorrhage or aneurysm originating from this artery. In 1868, Pilz reviewed 600 cases of carotid ligation, associated with a 43 percent mortality rate. In 1885, Victor Horsley was the first to perform this procedure for an intracranial aneurysm (Figure 8.4).

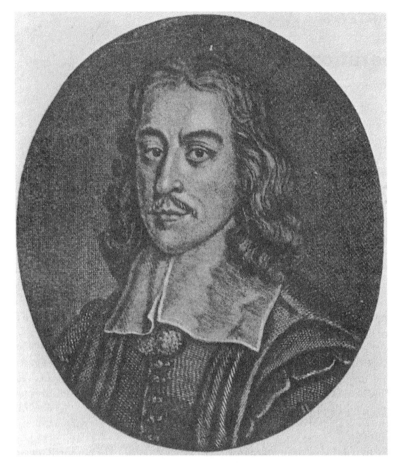

**Figure 8.1** Thomas Willis (from Garrison FH. *History of Medicine*. Philadelphia: WB Saunders Co., 1929).

It was widely accepted at the turn of the 20th century that the major cause of stroke was intracranial vascular disease, which was unamenable to therapy. This notion prevailed despite the report of Chiari in 1905, describing particles that could dislodge from an ulcerative plaque in the carotid vessels, resulting in stroke.

Ramsay Hunt, a neurologist at Columbia University, also played a major role in focusing attention on the carotid arteries as a possible source of cerebral vascular accidents. In an address to the American Neurologic Association in 1913, he suggested that intracranial cerebral vascular lesions might not cause strokes, as was commonly believed, but could result from them. He urged his colleagues to examine routinely the carotid arteries in all patients, clinically and pathologically:

> It would, therefore, seem proper in all cases with cerebral symptoms of vascular origin, to examine the pulsation of the carotids in the neck as possibly throwing some light on

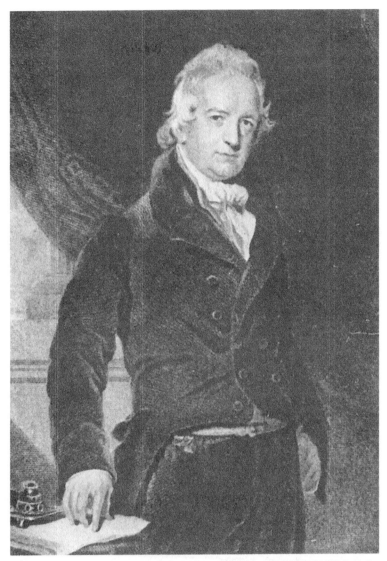

**Figure 8.2**  John Abernethy (from Garrison FH. *History of Medicine*. Philadelphia: WB Saunders Co., 1929).

the source of the obstruction and rendering more exact our localization of the seat of the trouble in this group of cases. For this purpose a section of the carotid artery is readily accessible to palpation, extending from the lower border of the thyroid cartilage to the angle of the jaw; the main trunk divides into the external and internal carotid at the level of the hyoid bone, and the internal, the larger of the two vessels, is readily felt from this point to the angle of the jaw.

In his discussion of hemiplegia associated with diminished carotid pulsations he stated:

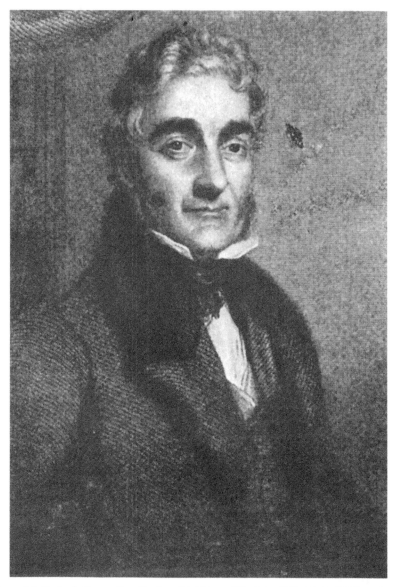

**Figure 8.3**  Benjamin Travers (from Garrison FH. *History of Medicine*. Philadelphia: WB Saunders Co., 1929).

While inequality of pulsation on the two sides might be accidental, its occurrence in four cases all presenting the symptoms of extensive brain softening is rather significant, and the thought naturally arises that some obstructive lesion of the vessel or its entrance into the arch of the aorta has interfered with the free flow of blood to the brain, which in old subjects with weakened heart would be a predisposing factor in the production of senile softening of the brain . . . . I would urge that in all cases presenting cerebral symptoms of vascular origin, that the main arteries of the neck be

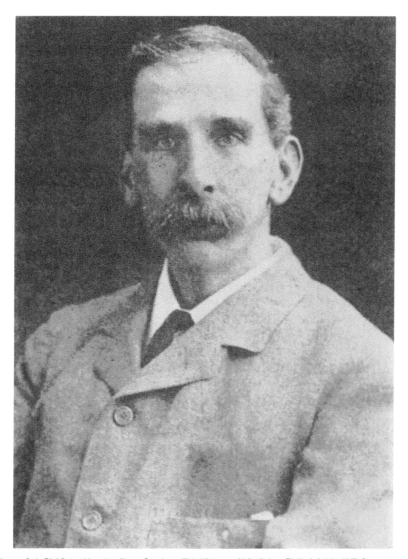

**Figure 8.4** Sir Victor Horsley (from Garrison FH. *History of Medicine*. Philadelphia: WB Saunders Co., 1929).

carefully examined for the possible diminution or absence of pulsation. Obstructive lesions of these vessels are apparently rare, but it seems certain that cases are overlooked from failure to make clinical and pathological examinations from this point of view.

A practical way of diagnosing carotid arterial occlusive disease was now required. In 1927, Egas Moniz of Lisbon described his technique of cerebral angiography as a method for localizing cerebral tumors (Figures 8.5 and 8.6). Ten years later, he reported the results of 537 cerebral angiograms in *Presse Médicale*. Four cases of internal carotid occlusion were noted. One year earlier, in

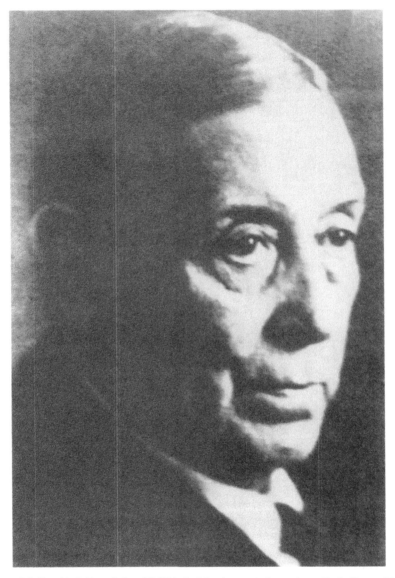

**Figure 8.5** Egas Moriz (from Callow AD. Historical development of vascular grafts. In: Sawyer PN, Kaplitt MJ, eds. *Vascular Grafts*. New York: Appleton-Century-Crofts, 1978).

1936, Sjoqvist had reported the first case of carotid occlusion demonstrated angiographically.

An important link between the contributions of Ramsay Hunt and the advent of carotid arterial reconstruction was provided in 1950 by Miller Fisher, a Canadian neurologist working at the Massachusetts General Hospital. He had performed 373 postmortem examinations of brains from patients who had died

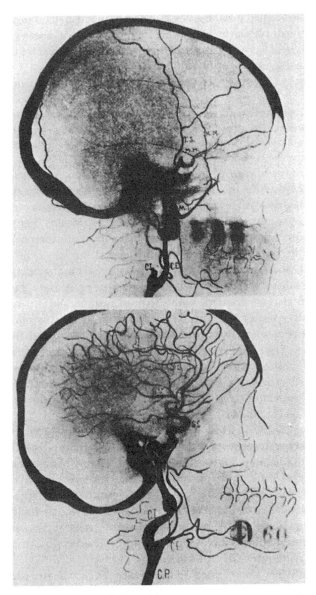

**Figure 8.6** Demonstration of internal carotid occlusion (top) and stenosis (bottom) by Moniz in two of his early cerebral angiograms (from Eastcott HHG, Pickering GW, Rob C. Reconstruction of internal carotid artery in a patient with intermittent attacks of hemiplegia. *Lancet* 1954; 2:994).

with a diagnosis of cerebral vascular occlusive disease. In an address to the American Association of Neuropathologists, Fisher reported that hemorrhagic infarcts were present in fewer than 20 percent of his specimens and concluded that most cases of stroke were embolic in origin. Fisher reaffirmed Hunt's earlier descriptions of atherosclerotic lesions at the carotid bifurcation, with partial or complete occlusion of these vessels. He also noted that the vessels distal to a stenosis at the carotid bifurcation were frequently free of disease. Fisher concluded: "No case of vascular disease of the brain is completely investigated if the carotid arteries have not been investigated."

Fisher inspired the first successful carotid arterial reconstruction when he wrote:

> . . . it is even conceivable that some day vascular surgery will find a way to by-pass the occluded portion of the artery during the period of ominous fleeting symptoms. Anastomosis of the external carotid artery, or one of its branches, with the internal carotid artery above the area of narrowing should be feasible.

The present era of carotid arterial reconstructive surgery began in Buenos Aires. It is doubtful that the names of any of the three Argentinean physicians involved in the first case of carotid revascularization would be recognized by many vascular surgeons today. Raul Carrea, Mahelz Molins (Figure 8.7), and Guillermo Murphy admitted a 41-year-old man who had suffered recent aphasia and a right hemiparesis to their neurosurgical service at the Institute of Experimental Medicine in September 1951. A cerebral angiogram performed 6 days later revealed a severe left internal carotid artery stenosis. One week later, the examination was repeated, with identical results. On October 20, 1951, Carrea partially resected the diseased portion of the internal carotid artery and performed an end-to-end anastomosis between the external and distal internal carotid arteries. The patient made an uneventful recovery and, after 39 months of follow-up, had a neurologic examination in which results were normal. Carrea referred to his technique as carotid–carotideal anastomosis, gave credit to Fisher for the idea, and concluded that it appeared to be the ideal treatment for carotid stenosis (Figure 8.8).

On January 28, 1953, Strully, Hurwitt, and Blankenberg attempted the first thromboendarterectomy of the internal carotid artery (Figure 8.8). Their patient was a 52-year-old man with recurrent left-sided cerebral hemispheric transient ischemic attacks. Angiograms performed 5 and 2 days earlier had revealed occlusion of the internal carotid artery. Despite removal of a large amount of thrombus, they were unable to achieve retrograde flow. Among their conclusions they maintained: "A by-passing arterial anastomosis or thromboendarterectomy should be successful when the occlusion is localized to the cervical portion of the internal carotid artery."

During the 1950s, many "firsts" in the history of vascular surgery took place in Houston, Texas. Among these was the first successful thromboendarterectomy of the carotid artery, performed by Michael DeBakey (Figure 8.8). His patient was a 53-year-old male bus driver with a 30-month history of left-sided cerebral hemispheric transient ischemic attacks. DeBakey reasoned that, since endarterectomy and graft replacement in other arteries could be performed, the carotid should not be an exception. DeBakey informed his patient that the surgical risk was slight and that if the operation did not correct his condition it probably would not change it. On August 7, 1953, a thromboendarterectomy of the common and internal carotid arteries was performed. An intraoperative arteri-

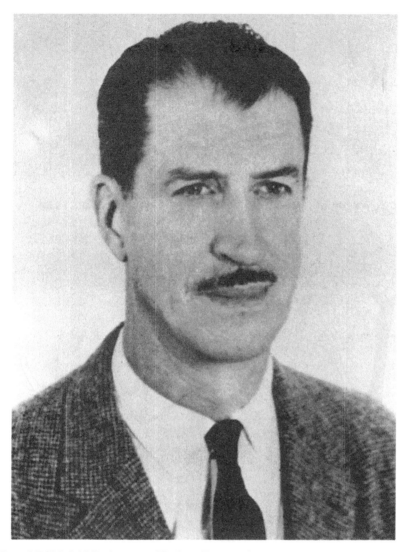

**Figure 8.7** Mahelz Molins (courtesy of Dr. Jesse Thompson).

ogram confirmed patency of the internal carotid artery. The arteriotomy was closed primarily with silk suture and the patient recovered uneventfully. He was discharged 8 days later and survived until 1972, without recurrence of neurologic symptoms. DeBakey reported this historic operation, as well as the 19-year follow-up, in the *Journal of the American Medical Association* in 1975. He concluded that such gratifying results provided encouragement for further application of this surgery.

Although it took place across the Atlantic 9 months after DeBakey's operation, the procedure performed by Eastcott, Pickering, and Rob was even more

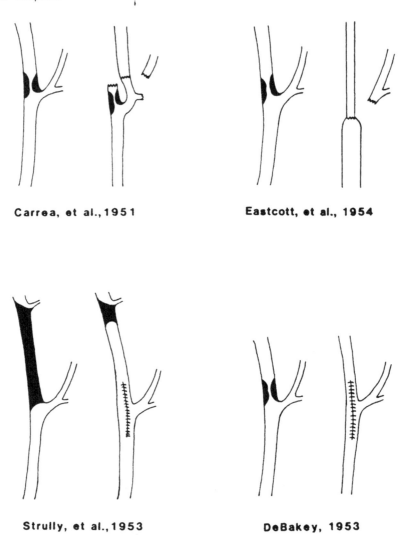

Carrea, et al., 1951          Eastcott, et al., 1954

Strully, et al., 1953          DeBakey, 1953

**Figure 8.8** The first carotid artery reconstructions.

influential in the development of carotid reconstructive surgery (Figure 8.8). Their patient was a 66-year-old housewife who had suffered 33 left-sided cerebral hemispheric and retinal transient attacks. An arteriogram revealed near occlusion of the left internal carotid artery. On May 19, 1954, the patient was taken to the operating room where her body temperature was reduced to 28°C by external cooling. She underwent resection of the left carotid bifurcation with end-to-end anastomosis of the common and internal carotid arteries. The patient made an uneventful recovery and was discharged 2 weeks later. Twenty years after her surgery, she remained free of symptoms.

Other initial attempts at carotid reconstruction included the first carotid resection with homograft replacement, performed in July 1954 by Denman. His patient was a 49-year-old man with symptomatic occlusion of both internal carotid arteries who underwent staged replacement of the carotid bifurcations with arterial homografts. In December 1955, Lin replaced a diseased carotid bifurcation with a 3-inch saphenous vein interposition graft in a 44-year-old man. The first subclavian–carotid bypass was performed by Lyons in August 1956 with a nylon prosthesis.

During the next several decades, the popularity of carotid endarterectomy soared. By 1984, over 100 000 of these procedures were being performed annually in the United States. In 1986, however, the annual increase in the number of patients undergoing carotid endarterectomy came to an abrupt halt. Carotid endarterectomy came under intense scrutiny for several reasons: there was a marked geographic variation in the performance of this operation throughout the United States, many unresolved questions about the appropriate indications for this surgery existed, and several reports of excessive morbidity and mortality in hospitals in the United States and in Europe appeared in the literature. The absence of a single rigorous clinical study demonstrating the efficacy of carotid endarterectomy was glaring. As a result of these questions, several large, multicenter, prospective, randomized trials were initiated. In 1991, when the number of carotid endarterectomies performed each year had declined to 70 000, the results of some of these studies appeared.

The current indications for carotid endarterectomy resulted from three trials that were reported in the 1990s. The North American Symptomatic Carotid Endarterectomy Trial (NASCET) sought to determine whether carotid endarterectomy reduced the risk of stroke in patients with a recent adverse cerebral vascular event and an ipsilateral carotid stenosis. It was conducted at 50 centers in the United States and Canada; 659 patients were enrolled. Life-table estimates of the cumulative risk of any ipsilateral stroke after 2 years were 26 percent in the 331 medical patients and 9 percent in the 328 surgical patients. For major or fatal ipsilateral strokes, the corresponding estimates were 13.1 percent and 2.5 percent respectively. The NASCET collaborators concluded that carotid endarterectomy was highly beneficial to patients with recent hemispheric and retinal transient ischemic attacks or to those with nondisabling strokes and ipsilateral high-grade stenosis.

The European Carotid Surgery Trial was another prospective, randomized, multicenter study that appeared in 1991. In the 778 patients with symptomatic, severe carotid stenosis, there was a significant reduction in the incidence of death and stroke after 3 years among patients who underwent carotid endarterectomy compared with nonoperative treatment (12.3 percent vs. 21.9 percent).

These trials, in addition to several smaller ones, provided reassurance that carotid endarterectomy was beneficial to patients with symptomatic lesions. The medical community waited 4 years for the results of the Asymptomatic Carotid Atherosclerosis Study (ACAS). This was also a prospective, randomized, multicenter trial across the United States and Canada. The results of 1659 patients with asymptomatic carotid artery stenosis of 60 percent or greater from 39 centers appeared in 1995. After a median follow-up of 2.7 years, the aggregate risk over 5 years for ipsilateral stroke and perioperative stroke or death was estimated to be 5.1 percent in surgical patients and 11 percent in medically treated patients. In the year that these results were published, approximately 130 000 endarterectomies were performed in the United States. Carotid endarterectomy was vindicated, or so it seemed.

Mullan performed the first carotid angioplasty in 1980. His patient was a 35-year-old woman who had recently undergone balloon occlusion of the left internal carotid artery for a large cavernous sinus aneurysm. She subsequently complained of a pulsating noise in her right ear; angiography revealed a "web-like constriction" in the right internal carotid artery. Six months of aspirin therapy had no effect on the symptoms, and a repeat angiogram revealed worsening of the internal carotid stenosis. Surgery was deemed too dangerous, and a Grüntzig dilating balloon was inflated eight times to remove the constriction. The patient's symptoms disappeared and the case was reported in the *Journal of Neurosurgery*.

In 1981, successful dilatation of internal carotid fibromuscular dysplastic lesions was achieved by Hasso and Garrido. A year later, Mathias also reported this feat.

The May/June 1983 issue of the *American Journal of Neuroradiology* contained three reports of percutaneous transluminal angioplasty of the internal carotid artery. Bockenheimer reported three cases of dilatation of arteriosclerotic lesions, with one complication; Wiggli reported successful dilatation of carotid lesions in two patients; and Tievsky reported successful dilatation of a postsurgical common carotid stenosis.

In 1984, Namaguchi also performed carotid angioplasty for a postendarterectomy stenosis, and by the end of the decade some practitioners were hailing carotid angioplasty as a superior alternative to endarterectomy. The initial results of carotid angioplasty did not support this claim.

The results of the first multicenter prospective study of carotid angioplasty appeared in 1993. The North American Percutaneous Transluminal Angioplasty Register (NACPTAR) described 165 angioplasties in 147 symptomatic patients. The immediate success rate was 83 percent, with a combined 30-day stroke and mortality rate of 9 percent.

In 1996, Roubin reported the results of another prospective study of 238 carotid angioplasties (61 percent for symptoms) in 204 patients. The mortality was 0.5 percent, the major stroke rate was 1 percent, and the minor stroke rate was 7.4 percent.

In 1996, the results of the Carotid and Vertebral Artery Transluminal Angioplasty Study (CAVATAS) were also reported. In this European prospective randomized comparison between carotid angioplasty and endarterectomy, the stroke and mortality rates among 504 patients were nearly identical.

With increasing operator experience and the introduction of distal protection devices, the reported results of carotid angioplasty improved in the late 1990s.

These facts, combined with the obvious appeal of avoiding a neck dissection, resulted in the Carotid Revascularization Endarterectomy Versus Stent Trial (CREST).

CREST is a multicenter, randomized, clinical trial, funded by the National Institute of Neurologic Disorders and Stroke (NINDS), of the National Institute of Health (NIH). The efficacy of carotid angioplasty versus endarterectomy in symptomatic patients with amaurosis fugax, transient ischemic attacks, or nondisabling strokes, associated with stenoses > 50 percent, will be evaluated. The incidence of stroke, myocardial infarction, and death within 30 days of intervention, and the incidence of ipsilateral stroke after 30 days, will be recorded. A sample size of 2500 will be sought, and it is hoped that definite clinical recommendations will be established based on this study.

## Bibliography

Bockenheimer SAM, Mathias K. Percutaneous transluminal angioplasty in arteriosclerotic internal carotid artery stenosis. *AJNR* 1983; 4:791.

Brott T, Thalinger K. The practice of carotid endarterectomy in a large metropolitan area. *Stroke* 1984; 15:959.

Carrea R, Molins M, Murphy G. Surgical treatment of spontaneous thrombosis of the internal carotid artery in the neck. Carotid-carotideal anastomosis. Report of a case. *Acta Neurol Latinoamer* 1955; 1:17.

Chassin MR, Brook RH, Park RE, *et al*. Variations in the use of medical and surgical services by the Medicare population. *N Engl J Med* 1986; 314:285.

Chiari H. Ueber das verhalten des teilungswinkels der carotis communis bei der endarteriitis chronica deformans. *Verh Dtsch Ges Pathol* 1905; 9:326.

Cooper AP. A case of aneurism of the carotid artery. *Tr Med-Chir Soc Edinburgh* 1809; 1:1.

Cooper AP. Account of the first successful operation performed on the common carotid artery for aneurysm in the year 1808 with the postmortem examination in the year 1821. *Guy Hosp Rep* 1836; 1:53.

DeBakey ME. Successful carotid endarterectomy for cerebrovascular insufficiency. Nineteen-year followup. *JAMA* 1975; 233:1083.

Denman FR, Ehni G, Duty WS. Insidious thrombotic occulsion of cervical carotid arteries, treated by arterial graft, a case report. *Surgery* 1955; 38:569.

Eastcott HHG, Pickering GW, Rob C. Reconstruction of internal carotid artery in a patient with intermittent attacks of hemiplegia. *Lancet* 1954; 2:994.

European Carotid Trialists' Collaborative Group. MCR European Carotid Surgery Trial: interim results for symptomatic patients with severe (70–99%) or with mild (0–29%) carotid stenosis. *Lancet* 1991; 337:1235.

Executive Committee for the Asymptomatic Carotid Atherosclerosis Study. Endarterectomy for asymptomatic carotid stenosis. *JAMA* 1995; 273:1421.

Fisher M. Occlusion of the internal carotid artery. *Arch Neurol Psychiat* 1951; 65:346.

Fisher M, Adams RD. Observation on brain embolism with special reference to the mechanism of hemorrhagic infarction. *J Neuropath Exp Neurol* 1951; 10:92.

Garrido E, Montoya J. Transluminal dilatation of internal carotid artery in fibromuscular dysplasia. *Surg Neurol* 1981; 16:469.

Hamby WB. *Intracranial Aneurysms*. Springfield: Charles C. Thomas, 1952.

Hasso AN, Bird CR, Zinke DE, et al. Fibromuscular dysplasia of the internal carotid artery: percutaneous transluminal angioplasty. *AJNR* 1981; 2:175.

Hobson RW, Ferguson R. Status report on the carotid revascularization endarterectomy versus stent trial. *Tech Vasc Interv Radiol* 2000; 3:1.

Hunt JR. The role of the carotid arteries, in the causation of vascular lesions on the brain, with remarks on certain special features of the symptomatology. *Am J Med Sci* 1914; 147:704.

Keen WW. Intracranial lesions. *Med News, NY* 1890; 57:443.

Lin PM, Javid H, Doyle EJ. Partial internal carotid artery occlusion treated by primary resection and vein graft. *J Neurosurg* 1956; 13:650.

Lyons C, Galbraith G. Surgical treatment of atherosclerotic occlusion of the internal carotid artery. *Ann Surg* 1957; 146:487.

Major ongoing stroke trials. Carotid and vertebral artery transluminal angioplasty study (CAVATAS). *Stroke* 1996; 27:358.

Mathias K, Heiss HW, Gospos C. Subclavian-steal-syndrom-operierien oder dilatieren? *Langenbecks Arch Chir* 1982; 356:279.

Mayberg MR, Wilson SE, Yatsu F, and the VA Symptomatic Carotid Stenosis Group. Carotid endarterectomy and prevention of cerebral ischemia in symptomatic carotid stenosis. *JAMA* 1991; 266:3289.

Moniz E. L'encéphalographie artérielle. Son importance dans la localisation des tumeurs cérébrales. *Rev Neurol* 1927; 2:72.

Moniz E, Lima A, de Lacerda R. Hémiplégies par thrombose de la carotide interne. *Presse Med* 1937; 45:977.

Mullan S, Duda EE, Patronas NJ. Some examples of balloon technology in neurosurgery. *J Neurosurg* 1980; 52:321.

Muuronen O. Outcome of surgical treatment of 110 patients with transient ischemic attack. *Stroke* 1984; 15:950.

NACPTAR (The North American Percutaneous Transluminal Angioplasty Register) Investigators. Update of the immediate angiographic results and in-hospital central nervous system complications of cerebral percutaneous transluminal angioplasty. *Circulation* 1995; 92:1.

NACPTAR (The North American Percutaneous Transluminal Angioplasty Register) Investigators. Restenosis following cerebral percutaneous transluminal angioplasty. *Stroke* 1995; 26:186.

Namaguchi Y, Puyau FA, Provenza LJ, et al. Percutaneous transluminal angioplasty of the carotid artery: its application to post surgical stenosis. *Neuroradiology* 1984; 26:527.

North American Symptomatic Carotid Endarterectomy Trial Collaborators. Beneficial effect of carotid endarterectomy in symptomatic patients with high-grade carotid stenosis. *N Engl J Med* 1991; 325:445.

Paré A. *The Workes of that Famous Chirurgion Ambroise Parey: Translated out of Latine and Compared with the French, by Thomas Johnson. 1634.* New York: Milford House, Inc, 1968.

Pilz C. Zur ligatur der arteria carotis communis, nebst einer statistik dieser operation. *Arch Klin Chir* 1868; 9:257.

Roubin GS, Yadav S, Iyes SS, et al. Carotid stent-supported angioplasty: a neurovascular intervention to prevent stroke. *Am J Cardiol* 1996; 78:8.

Sjoqvist O. Ueber intrakranielle aneurysmen der arteria carotis und deren beziehung zur ophthalmoplegischen migraine. *Nervenarzt* 1936; 9:233.

Strully KJ, Hurwitt ES, Blankenberg HW. Thrombo-endarterectomy for thrombosis of the internal carotid artery in the neck. *J Neurosurg* 1953; 10:474.

Symonds C. The circle of Willis. *Br Med J* 1955; 1:119.

Tievsky AL, Druy EM, Mardiat JG. Transluminal angioplasty in postsurgical stenosis of the extracranial carotid artery. *AJNR* 1983; 40:800.

Travers B. A case of aneurism by anastomosis in the orbit, cured by ligation of the common carotid artery. *Med Chir Tr* 1811; 2:1.

Tu JV, Hannan EL, Anderson GM, *et al*. The fall and rise of carotid endarterectomy in the United States and Canada. *N Engl J Med* 1998; 339:1441.

Warlow C. Carotid endarterectomy: does it work? *Stroke* 1984; 15:1068.

Wiggli U, Gratzl O. Transluminal angioplasty of stenotic carotid arteries: case reports and protocol. *AJNR* 1983; 49:793.

PART 4

# Yankee ingenuity

# CHAPTER 9

# Valentine Mott

*Courage is not simply one of the virtues, but the form of every virtue at the testing point.*

*(C.S. Lewis)*

Mott was born in Glen Cove, New York, in 1785 (Figure 9.1). His father, Henry, was a physician of English descent with a strong Quaker background. The Mott family moved to Newton, New York, when Valentine was 6 years old. Mott attended a private seminary there until the age of 19.

Mott never attended college and began medical studies with his cousin Valentine Seaman, a New York City surgeon. He also began attending medical lectures at Columbia College.

In 1806, Mott received his medical degree, then spent an additional year studying with Seaman. Mott's tutelage under his cousin affected him significantly and Mott decided to travel abroad for further surgical training.

In the early 19th century, Astley Cooper was the most renowned surgical educator in Europe. Americans wanting the best surgical training strived to enroll at Guy's Hospital in London. Mott traveled there in 1807 and soon became Cooper's wound dresser, thanks largely to the fine job John Warren had performed 7 years earlier. The 6 months that Mott spent with Cooper profoundly influenced his approach to surgical problems. Mott had tremendous respect and admiration for the skills of his legendary teacher, particularly after he witnessed the operation performed on Humphrey Humphreys for a carotid aneurysm. After his apprenticeship with Cooper, Mott spent an additional year studying with several other great English surgeons: John Abernethy, Henry Cline, William Blizzard, and Evevard Home.

Mott returned to New York in 1809 and began to conduct private lessons in surgery. He had the styles of all the great English surgeons to draw upon, and his fame as a teacher grew quickly. One year later, he became a Lecturer on Surgery and Demonstrator in Anatomy at Columbia College. Mott was proud of his teaching ability and endeavored to impart the principles of surgery in as scientific and systematic a way as his mentor, Astley Cooper, had done. In 1811, Mott became Professor of Surgery and he continued to enjoy increasing popularity as a teacher.

In 1813, the Columbia College merged with the College of Physicians and Surgeons in New York, and Mott became the first Chairman of Surgery in the new school. During his fourth year in this position, he was asked to see a patient with a subclavian artery aneurysm. Like Cooper, Mott performed the first of several original operations when he ligated the patient's innominate artery. The patient survived for nearly 1 month, but eventually exsanguinated following necrosis of the aneurysm. Although saddened by the outcome of the case, Mott

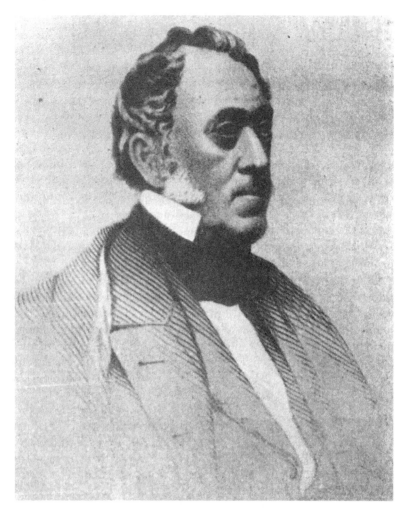

**Figure 9.1** Valentine Mott (from Major RA. *A History of Medicine.* Springfield, IL: Charles C Thomas, 1954).

felt justified in performing the operation and considered it a major contribution to surgery. The ultimate praise was offered by Astley Cooper who, upon learning of the procedure, stated, "I would rather be the author of that one operation than of all I have ever originated."

In 1821 and 1824, Mott performed two other operations that further enhanced his reputation. The first patient had an osteosarcoma of the mandible for which Mott performed ligation of the carotid artery and mandibulectomy (Figure 9.2). In an age without anesthesia, blood replacement, and antisepsis, this operation was a great feat. Mott's second case involved a 10-year-old boy who suffered nonunion of a femur fracture. In this case, Mott performed the first successful hip disarticulation in the United States (Figure 9.3).

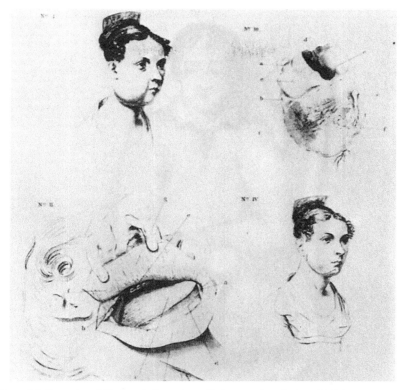

**Figure 9.2** Illustration of Mott's technique of mandibulectomy (from Rutkow IM. Valentine Mott (1785–1865), the father of American vascular surgery: A historical perspective. *Surgery* 1979; 85:441).

In 1826, the entire medical faculty of the College of Physicians and Surgeons resigned over a political dispute with the hospital trustees. These disgruntled physicians created a separate New York Medical College, which operated under the auspices of Rutgers College in New Jersey. As a result of legal difficulties, this arrangement ceased within 5 years, but it gave Mott the opportunity to perform several more original operations.

The first was ligation of the common iliac artery just distal to the aortic bifurcation, for an aneurysm of the external iliac artery. Mott performed this procedure in less than an hour. At Rutgers, Mott also carried out the first clavicular excision for an osteosarcoma involving the adjacent subclavian and jugular veins. The procedure took 4 hours to complete and at one point during the procedure the patient was in hemorrhagic shock. Mott was shaken by this operation and noted:

> . . . this operation far surpassed in tediousness, difficulty and danger, anything which I have ever witnessed or performed. It is impossible for any description which we are capable of giving, to convey an accurate idea of its formidable nature.

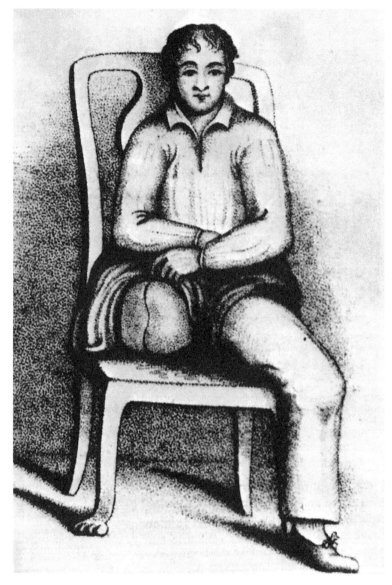

**Figure 9.3** Patient following hip disarticulation performed by Mott (from Rutkow IM. Valentine Mott (1785–1865), the father of American vascular surgery: A historical perspective. *Surgery* 1979; 85:441).

Mott later described this procedure as the most difficult operation that can be performed in man.

By 1834, Mott's heavy schedule had exacted a toll on his health. He retired as Chief of Surgery in order to return to Europe and resume his travels. In February 1835, an honorary public dinner was held for Mott.

It is no surprise that Mott's first stop in Europe was a visit with Astley Cooper. It had been 25 years since Cooper had seen his prized pupil. Cooper was delighted at the chance to discuss old times and he presented Mott with a set of personally designed surgical instruments when the two great surgeons bade each other farewell.

Mott's travels continued for 6 more years through Europe, taking him as far as Africa. He visited Ireland, Great Britain, Belgium, France, Holland, Germany, Greece, Italy, Turkey, and Egypt. During this time, he remained in touch with friends and family in New York; he returned home in 1841.

Rejuvenated by his journey, Mott agreed to become the Chairman of Surgery at the New York University Medical College. Over the next 10 years, he again developed a large practice and authored several more original operations.

Mott's health began to fail again in 1850; 3 years later he retired and accepted an emeritus position. He continued to teach and occasionally to operate. During the Civil War, Mott was active in aiding the wounded. In 1862, he reported two studies regarding the treatment of bleeding wounds and the use of anesthetics.

Toward the end of his life, Mott suffered increasingly from angina. He died on April 15, 1865, 2 days after the assassination of Abraham Lincoln. Mott had a gangrenous leg and his feeble health precluded consideration of amputation.

A review of Mott's surgical record reveals how remarkable he was for his time. It included ligation of one innominate artery, eight subclavian arteries, two common carotid, 51 external carotid, one common iliac, six external iliac, two internal iliac, 57 femoral, and 10 popliteal arteries. The fact that Mott worked without benefit of transfusions, anesthesia, or antiseptics makes his record even more impressive.

Mott also performed 165 lithotomies and over 900 amputations. Valentine Mott brought the teachings and principles of John Hunter and Astley Cooper to the New World and elevated surgery to an accepted science in the United States.

## Bibliography

Anon. Valentine Mott—A great American surgeon and his association with Guy's Hospital. *Guy's Hospital Rep* 1945; 94:75.

Bush RB, Bush IM. Valentine Mott (1785–1865). *Invest Urol* 1974; 12:162.

Rutkow IM. Valentine Mott (1785–1865), the father of American vascular surgery: A historical perspective. *Surgery* 1979; 85:441.

# CHAPTER 10

# Rudolph Matas

*If a man will begin with certainties, he shall end in doubts; but if he will be content to begin with doubts he shall end in certainties.*

(Francis Bacon)

A significant portion of the history of vascular surgery can be traced by studying the evolution of the treatment of aneurysms. Some of the greatest contributions to treatment of these lesions were made by Rudolph Matas (Figure 10.1). He operated on more than 600 aneurysms, with remarkably low complication and death rates. Through his pioneering efforts successful treatment of aneurysms became commonplace, and Matas became one of the preeminent figures in vascular surgery.

Rudolph Matas was born on September 11, 1860, on a Louisiana plantation, Bonnet Carre. His parents had emigrated from Europe 4 years earlier. Matas's father, Narciso, had earned a doctorate degree in pharmacy in 1858, and one in medicine at the New Orleans College of Medicine during the following year. After receiving the second degree, Narciso served as plantation physician at Bonnet Carre.

The elder Matas had formed an association with some of the cotton speculators and other traders in New Orleans during the federal occupation of Louisiana. While the precise nature of his business dealings is not completely clear, he did profit substantially. In 1863, he was forced to move abroad temporarily. The family left for Paris, where Narciso studied ophthalmology. Rudolph became familiar with the anatomy of the eye, a taunting irony since severe problems with his own eyes would result in enucleation of one and near blindness in the other toward the end of his life.

As a child, the younger Matas also learned to speak French, Spanish, and Catalan. Rudolph suffered numerous interruptions in his early education as moves to Barcelona, back to New Orleans in 1867, and to Brownsville, Texas, followed the years in Paris. He then spent 1 year in a Spanish parochial school in Matamoros, followed by 2 years in a New Orleans parochial school.

Matas next entered the St. John's Collegiate Institute in Matamoros and graduated in 1877. He was accepted to the Medical Department of the University of Louisiana, which would later become Tulane University. Matas earned his MD degree in 1880, before the age of 20.

During the next 2 years, Matas was a resident at Charity Hospital in New Orleans, after which he went into private practice. While in that practice, Matas served as a surgery and anatomy instructor at Charity Hospital.

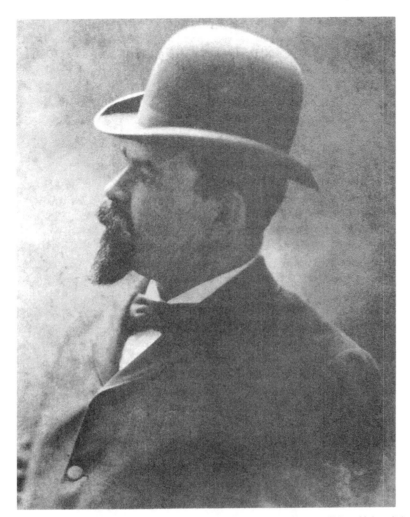

**Figure 10.1** Rudolph Matas (courtesy of the Howard-Tilton Memorial Library, Tulane University).

Matas could never have suspected that a 26-year-old plantation worker from St. Mary Parish would be responsible for his first steps on the road to surgical immortality. In January 1888, while rabbit hunting with some fellow workers, Manuel Harris sustained an accidental shotgun wound to his left upper arm. Two weeks later, he noted a pulsatile swelling between his elbow and axilla. In March 1888, after it continued to grown in size, he was admitted to Charity Hospital with a traumatic aneurysm of the brachial artery (Figure 10.2).

Matas met Harris on a hospital ward. Matas was initially loath to employ the usual treatment of extremity amputation, or proximal and distal arterial ligation, out of concern for his patient, who could only maintain his livelihood with two viable upper extremities. Matas, therefore, attempted to thrombose the aneurysm using an Esmarch tourniquet, as well as digital and mechanical

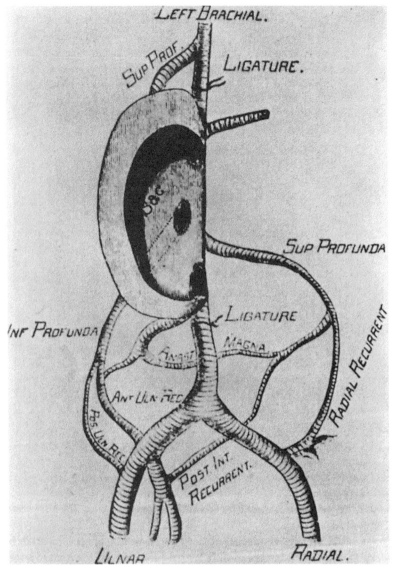

**Figure 10.2** Matas's illustration of Manuel Harris's aneurysm (from Matas R. Traumatic aneurysm of the left brachial artery. *Med News Phil* 1888; 53:462).

compression. So hesitant was Matas to operate on Harris that he employed this treatment for nearly 3 weeks. When each of these failed, he declared: "... we will have to empty this sac or dissect it right out of his arm."

On April 23, Matas performed proximal ligation of the brachial artery to treat the aneurysm. The pulsations were initially arrested, but on May 2 they returned. On May 3, Matas unsuccessfully attempted distal ligation. Only then did Matas open the aneurysm sac and, mindful of the neighboring vital structures, perform the endoaneurysmorrhaphy technique for which he became famous. All the while he credited Antyllus, who had performed this operation almost 18 centuries earlier.

Manuel Harris recovered rapidly from his surgery and left the hospital on May 21 with a functional arm. In 1898, Matas accidentally saw his patient again and observed that he was gainfully employed, with a palpable radial pulse. Although Matas had several opportunities to repeat this new procedure he could not ". . . muster sufficient courage to battle against tradition" and did not attempt this technique again until 1900.

Matas's ingenuity led him to develop various treatments for the different types of aneurysms that he encountered. He eventually described three forms of aneurysmorrhaphy: obliterative, restorative, and reconstructive. In the first, sutures from within the aneurysm sac were used to completely occlude branches arising from it, as well as the proximal and distal artery. The latter two were modifications of the obliterative type and allowed preservation of arterial patency. Matas would place a catheter into the main arteries and obliterate the sac over the catheter with sutures. He called this technique endoaneurysmorrhaphy with partial or complete arterioplasty. By successfully operating on many aneurysms, Matas demonstrated the efficacy of a direct surgical approach and encouraged others to pursue this form of treatment. Matas's general technique of endoaneurysmorrhaphy is employed by all vascular surgeons today.

In 1895, Matas was appointed professor and Chief of the Department of Surgery at Tulane University. He would hold this post for 32 years. In 1927, he became Emeritus Professor.

In 1900, Matas attempted to treat an abdominal aortic aneurysm by introducing wire and an electric current into it. Undaunted by the failure of this technique, he sought different ways to treat these lesions.

In 1923, Matas ligated the infrarenal aorta proximal to a large aneurysm, with survival of his patient. This was the first successful use of proximal ligation for an abdominal aortic aneurysm.

In 1908, Matas's career was threatened when he developed an infection of the right eye following surgery on a patient with a gonorrheal pelvic infection. Matas developed glaucoma, with eventual destruction of the iris and cornea. After nearly 4 months of severe pain from the effects of the infection, Matas underwent enucleation. He endured this discomfiting affliction for so long because he worried that the loss of binocular vision would interfere with his ability to operate. Matas was sensitive about the loss of his eye and shunned public appearances until an artificial one had been made. When photographed, he would always turn his head to the right, rendering it less noticeable. Matas was relieved following the loss of his eye when he noted little diminution of his operating ability. His good humor and talent as a writer were evident in a letter he wrote to a friend who had also suffered the loss of an eye:

> I am pleased to state in spite of the additional handicap of a marked myopea and astigmatism in my remaining eye, I have never done more minute and exacting work than

in the seven years that have elapsed since the accident which deprived me of my right and best eye.... My heartfelt congratulations on your splendid recovery – a recovery which will permit us, the cyclopeans, to enjoy the privilege of your conspicuous and inspiring example as a member of our band, just as the Binoculars have been honored by your leadership in the past.

In 1940, Matas reported his personal experience with the treatment of aneurysms to the American Surgical Association. It consisted of 620 operations. Of these, 101 were variations of his endoaneurysmorrhaphy technique. One of the most remarkable aspects of this experience was the mortality rate of less than 5 percent. In addition, none of the procedures resulted in gangrene.

Matas remained active in writing and teaching well into his nineties. He achieved an international reputation for his contributions to general and vascular surgery. One of his most famous lectures was entitled "The Soul of the Surgeon." Matas presented it to the Mississippi State Medical Society in 1915 and it revealed his great thoughtfulness and sensitivity.

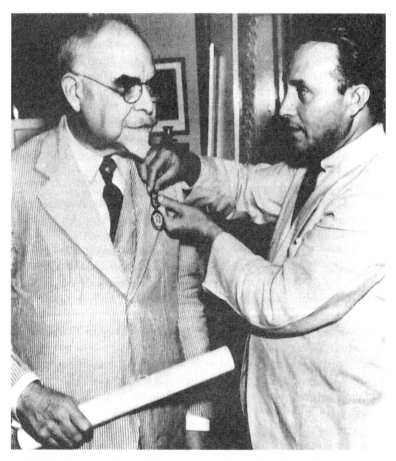

**Figure 10.3** The Venezuelan Medal of Honor awarded to Matas in 1934 by their Consul General (courtesy of the Howard-Tilton Memorial Library, Tulane University).

Matas's admonitions are timely today as he warned of those who would disgrace their profession for money and fame, and of others who would allow their vanity to eclipse reason and morality. Matas condemned the practice of fee splitting, having years earlier helped form the American College of Surgeons to root out this and other egregious practices. Matas defined the soul of the surgeon as: "... the ethical and emotional part of man's nature, the seat of the sentiments and feelings, as distinguished from pure intellect." He felt that only another surgeon could truly appreciate these thoughts.

Like all great men in the history of vascular surgery, Matas's contributions

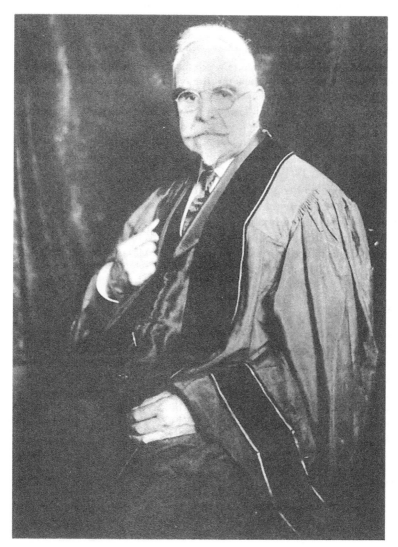

**Figure 10.4** Portrait of Matas by Thomas C. Corner (courtesy of the Howard-Tilton Memorial Library, Tulane University).

were not confined to this field. As a medical student, he had spent 3 months in Havana as a member of the Yellow Fever Commission, studying the mode of transmission of this disease. He was also an early supporter of surgical treatment for acute appendicitis and thyroidectomy for malignancy of the gland. Matas pioneered the intravenous use of saline solutions to treat hypovolemia and he encouraged the use of nasogastric and endotracheal tubes in surgery. He even reported the use of spinal anesthesia in 1900.

Matas was deeply saddened toward the end of this life when the vision in his left eye began to fail, secondary to glaucoma and cataract. In March 1952, at the age of 92, he underwent iridectomy and removal of the cataract. The operation failed, resulting in Matas's blindness. The darkness was particularly overwhelming since Matas's main joy was reading and corresponding with friends and colleagues. His unvanquished spirit, though somewhat weakened, was evident in another letter to a friend:

> I am still living in a world of shadows, which, though not seriously affecting my general health, has deprived me of practically all my visual efficiency. While no one can be very cheerful living in the penumbra of a ghost world, I am not rehearsing the lamentation of Job, and still manage to live in fairly good comfort, through the kindness and assistance of friends.

In January 1956, Matas was hospitalized owing to general weakness and inability to care for himself. He languished there for the remainder of his life and died on September 23, 1957, at the age of 97.

Matas embodied the greatest attributes of a physician. He was a renowned teacher, devoted scientist, and a dedicated humanitarian (Figures 10.3 and 10.4). One faithful student, Hermann Gessner, best reflected the high regard in which Matas was held when, as a student of Matas, he commented that he never needed any journals or textbooks: "I just attend all of Matas's operations and listen. Sooner or later I'll hear it all from him."

## Bibliography

Cohn I, Deutsch B. *Rudolph Matas: A Biography of One of the Great Pioneers in Surgery*. Garden City: Doubleday & Co, Inc, 1960.

Cordell AR. A lasting legacy: The life and work of Rudolph Matas. *J Vasc Surg* 1985; 2:613.

Creech O Jr. Rudolph Matas and Keen's surgery. *Am J Surg* 1967; 113:791.

Matas R. Traumatic aneurysm of the left brachial artery. *Med News Phil* 1888; 53:462.

Matas R. Treatment of abdominal aortic aneurysm by wiring and electrolysis. Critical study of the Moore-Corradi method based upon the latest clinical data. *Trans So Surg Assoc* 1900; 13:272.

Matas R. The soul of the surgeon. *Tr Miss M Assoc* 1915; 48:149.

Matas R. Ligation of the abdominal aorta. *Ann Surg* 1925; 81:457.

Matas R. Personal experiences in vascular surgery. A statistical synopsis. *Ann Surg* 1940; 112:802.

Shumacker HB Jr. A moment with Matas. *Surg Gynecol Obstet* 1977; 144:93.

# CHAPTER 11

# The arterial prosthesis: Arthur Voorhees

*One characteristic of American research is the cheerful optimism and a certain gay spirit of enterprise which animates the majority of scientists. They attack problems even when these offer slight prospect of solution, and when sensible people shake their heads. They try a shot and very frequently hit the mark.*

*(Henry Sigerist)*

Arthur Voorhees was born in Moorestown, New Jersey, in December 1921. His father, Arthur Sr., represented the tenth generation of the family in the United States, descended from Dutch farmers in Manhattan. Because the elder Voorhees had not taken full advantage of his education, he continually encouraged Arthur to seek advanced schooling. The two became very close and Voorhees looked to his father as a role model. He most admired his father's remarkable memory and great ability to "build better mouse traps."

Voorhees attended the Moorestown Friends' School. He did well scholastically and also starred in baseball and soccer. When the decision regarding an appropriate college needed to be made, Voorhees's mother was adamant that Arthur attend a southern university. A native of Jacksonville, Alabama, Mrs. Voorhees had never adjusted to the uncouth and indecorous ways of the North; she feared her son would be deprived of a proper education if he remained above the Mason–Dixon line. Thomas Jefferson had been a boyhood idol of Voorhees, so his choice to attend the University of Virginia in Charlottesville was a logical one.

Voorhees departed for the South in 1940 and had a rude awakening. The student body at the University of Virginia was competitive and Voorhees was no longer the standout he had been in high school. He recovered from a failing grade in French during his freshman year and went on to major in biology, with honors. He also excelled in physics and mathematics. Voorhees's maternal grandfather had been a country physician in Alabama and, again at his mother's urging, a career in medicine was determined for Arthur.

The bombing of Pearl Harbor occurred during Voorhees's second year in Virginia. Medical schools throughout the country accelerated their education programs and Voorhees, after applying to only one medical school, was accepted to Columbia University following his junior year of college.

Physicians and Surgeons was a frightening experience for Voorhees in 1943, particularly when he came close to failing anatomy (Figure 11.1). Some encouragement from his Dean and the Army's Specialized Training Corps advisor helped him to improve his grades (Figure 11.2).

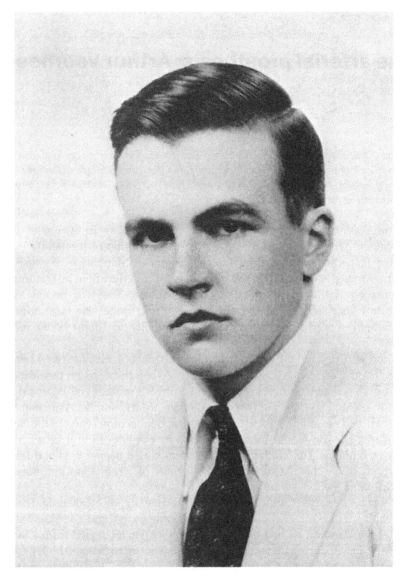

**Figure 11.1** Voorhees upon entrance into Physicians and Surgeons in 1943 (courtesy of Mrs. Margaret R. Voorhees).

After the first year of medical school, Voorhees was attracted to the "manual engineering" aspects of surgery. Working with Dr. Hugh Auchencloss during his second year at Columbia convinced Voorhees that surgery was the right field. Voorhees received his medical degree in 1946 and began his surgical internship. Following his internship, Arthur Blakemore offered Voorhees a research fellowship. It was the beginning of a long and fruitful association in

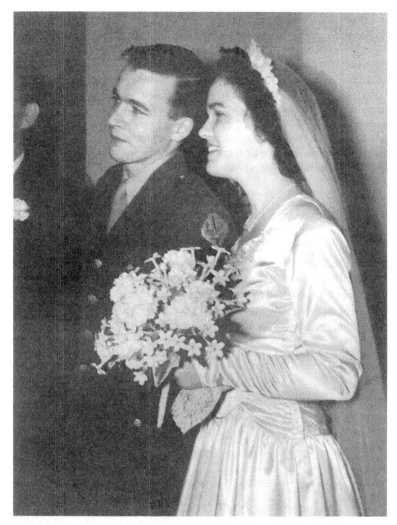

**Figure 11.2** Dr. and Mrs. Arthur Voorhees (courtesy of Mrs. Margaret R. Voorhees).

which, according to Voorhees: "Dr. Blakemore encouraged and supported my flight of medical and surgical fantasy."

It was during the fellowship year that Voorhees made a simple observation that would revolutionize the field of vascular surgery. Among other projects in the spring of 1947, Voorhees was working on a "bag valve" model for replacing the mitral valve, constructed from canine inferior vena cavas. The valves were stapled into the mitral annulus and silk sutures were used as chordae tendineae sewn full thickness into the ventricle of the beating animal heart. This was all performed through a left atrial pursestring. It is easy to imagine how in one animal Voorhees unwittingly misplaced a silk suture. He described the experiment in the following manner:

> During one of the early in vivo trials I made an error in placing the ventricular suture with the result that the stitch traversed the central part of the ventricular cavity. It would have been too difficult to correct but I did make a note of my error so that several months later, at autopsy, I took pains to find the misplaced suture. To my surprise it was coated with what grossly appeared to be endocardium. It resembled a normal chorda except for the black core of the stitch. It was a fragile structure which did not withstand microscopic sectioning, but its appearance was sufficiently startling to make me wonder if a piece of cloth might react in a similar way. From there I speculated that a cloth tube acting as a latticework of threads, might indeed serve as an arterial prosthesis.

Unknown to Voorhees, Guthrie had speculated about this possibility 30 years earlier, but had gone no further. Voorhees was aware of the tremendous possibilities inherent in these observations. He presented them to Blakemore, who was equally enthusiastic.

At a time when blood vessel banks were being developed throughout the country, Voorhees quickly gained proficiency on a sewing machine in order to manufacture an alternative to homografts (Figure 11.3). To test his idea, the first fabric prosthesis was a silk handkerchief fashioned into a tube and placed into the abdominal aorta of a dog. Voorhees used silk sutures for the anastomosis as

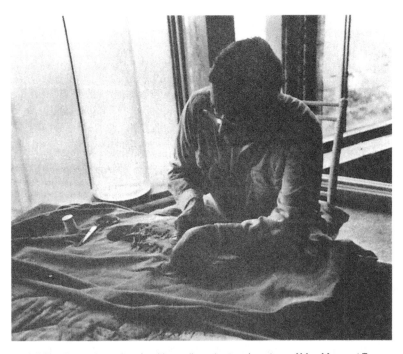

**Figure 11.3** Voorhees, always handy with needle and suture (courtesy of Mrs. Margaret R. Voorhees).

well. For 1 hour the graft remained patent, until the animal succumbed to a hemorrhage through the pores of the handkerchief prosthesis and anastomoses.

In 1948, Voorhees was assigned to the Brook Army Medical Center in San Antonio, Texas. Although his assigned task was to develop new and more effective plasma expanders, the excitement he felt after implanting a silk tube graft compelled him to continue his work on arterial substitutes. The Union Carbide Company generously donated a bolt of vinyon-N cloth, the material from which parachutes were manufactured. It was too inert to be dyed and, therefore, had little commercial value.

Voorhees continued to construct his grafts on sewing machines borrowed from neighbors, and while in Texas implanted six additional prostheses. A combination of hemorrhagic shock, excessive anesthesia, and the Texas heat was more than the experimental animals could tolerate, except for one dog that survived for a month. At autopsy, the graft was patent, albeit wrinkled and redundant. Upon returning to Columbia in 1950 to resume his surgical residency, Voorhees knew his idea would work.

Under the continued direction of Arthur Blakemore and John Lockwood, refinements were made in the construction and implantation of the vinyon-N grafts. Voorhees's colleagues in the Department of Pathology at Columbia played a key role in his understanding of graft healing. The microtomes at Brook had not been sharp enough to cut vinyon-N, consequently Voorhees had no histologic information until his return to New York. He soon realized that pore size was critical to the ingrowth of fibroblasts and that, without the latter, there could be no support for the neoendothelium. In addition, hematoma formation about the graft prevented proper healing. By the end of 1950, vinyon-N implants had been placed in approximately 40 dogs. Three-quarters of the animals survived the surgery for eventual autopsy study (Figure 11.4).

In 1951, Alfred Jaretzki joined the Voorhees–Blakemore team, and their first report of 15 animals with cloth prostheses appeared in the *Annals of Surgery* in March 1952.

The test in humans came several months later when an elderly man was brought into the emergency room at Columbia with a ruptured abdominal aortic aneurysm. The artery bank at New York Hospital was depleted and Voorhees raced to his laboratory one floor above the operating room, constructed a vinyon-N tube, and placed it in the autoclave. Although their patient was hemodynamically unstable, the graft was successfully implanted. It functioned for 30 minutes before the patient died from a myocardial infarction, secondary to hemorrhagic shock and coagulopathy.

Undaunted by this outcome, the group persisted with their work in humans. Their results were summarized by Voorhees in 1953 before the American Surgical Society in Cleveland, and in 1954 they reported the outcome of vinyon-N cloth tubes used to replace 17 abdominal aortic and one popliteal aneurysm. The surgical world received these reports with tremendous excitement. Laboratories were set up throughout the country to explore the use of different textiles and methods of fabrication. Union Carbide eventually ceased production of

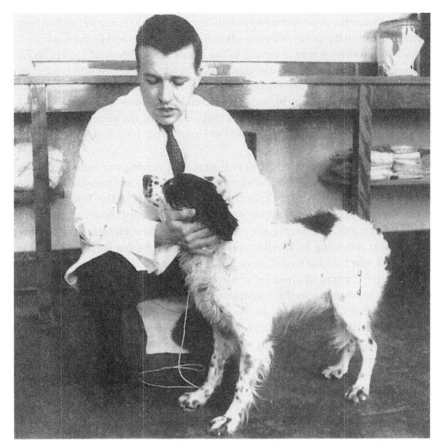

**Figure 11.4** Arthur Voorhees with the first survivor of implantation of aortic prosthesis (courtesy of Mrs. Margaret R. Voorhees).

vinyon-N and the use or Orlon, Teflon, nylon, and Dacron was investigated. Surgical meetings assumed the air of textile conventions, as surgeons readily adopted a new lexicon. Terms such as crimping, needle-per-inch ratio, and tuftal rhexis were glibly bandied about by these pioneers of prosthetic arterial replacement. Mass production of fabric prostheses soon followed, and with it the modern era of vascular surgery began.

Voorhees completed his surgical residency in 1955 and joined the faculty of Columbia-Presbyterian Hospital as an assistant attending surgeon (Figure 11.5). He was excited to continue working with Blakemore, and within 2 years they had implanted 50 Orlon grafts.

In addition to his pioneering work in vascular prosthetics, Voorhees also collaborated with Blakemore on refinement of the Sengstaken–Blakemore tube, and on the management of portal hypertension. In 1965, he reported the results of surgery for portal hypertension in 98 children; 8 years later he described

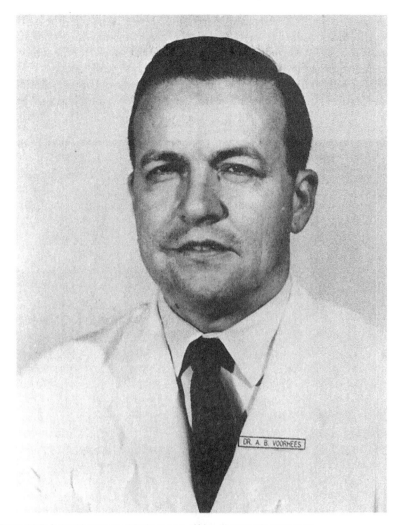

**Figure 11.5** Arthur Voorhees, 1956 (courtesy of Mrs. Margaret R. Voorhees).

the neurologic and psychiatric consequences of portal–systemic shunts in this population.

Voorhees became the director of the animal laboratory at Columbia after Blakemore retired. Voorhees soon had the laboratory renamed after his mentor, and important contributions in portal flow dynamics, hepatic regeneration, ammonia intoxication, and arterial substitutes continued to emanate from it.

In 1970, Voorhees became Professor of Surgery and Chief of the Vascular Surgery Service at Columbia. He held prominent positions in the New York Society of Cardiovascular Surgery and the North American Chapter of the International Society for Cardiovascular Surgery. Voorhees lectured throughout Europe and South America and eventually garnered the Lifetime Achievements in Medicine Award from the College of Physicians and Surgeons Alumni Association. In 1978, Voorhees initiated the Blakemore award for the senior surgical resident judged most productive in research during residency.

Voorhees retired from active practice in 1983 because of chronic pulmonary disease (Figure 11.6). He and his wife moved to West Stockbridge, in the

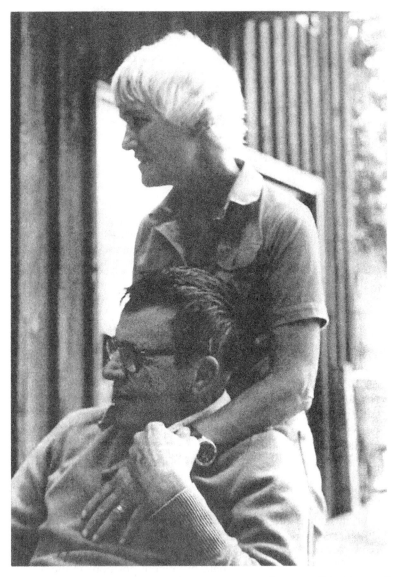

**Figure 11.6** Voorhees with wife Margaret, after retirement in 1984 (courtesy of Mrs. Margaret R. Voorhees).

Berkshire Mountains of Massachusetts (Figure 11.7). There, Voorhees enjoyed woodworking, gardening, birdwatching, and music. During the summers, the Voorheeses would visit a dude ranch in Arizona, where his breathing was less labored. In 1990, Albuquerque became their final home. Voorhees died on May 12, 1992, from a metastatic brain tumor.

Many scientific discoveries occur serendipitously and Voorhees's observation of canine endocardium growing onto a silk suture was such an event.

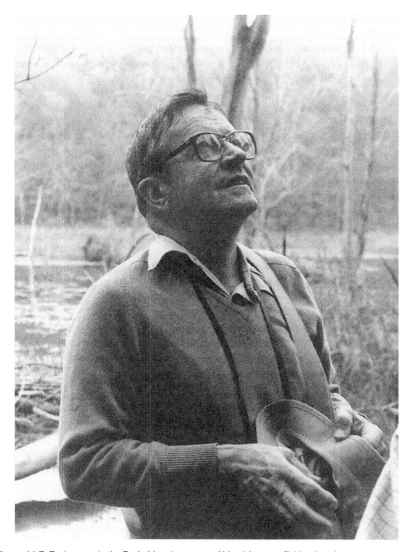

**Figure 11.7** Retirement in the Berkshires (courtesy of Mrs. Margaret R. Voorhees).

Voorhees was a vascular surgery pioneer in the United States and his innovation began a new era in the field.

## Bibliography

Blakemore AH, Voorhees AB Jr. The use of tubes constructed from vinyon "N" cloth in bridging arterial defects—experimental and clinical. *Ann Surg* 1954; 140:324.

Britton RC, Voorhees AB Jr., Price JB Jr. Selective portal decompression. *Surgery* 1970; 67:104.

Greisler HP, Kim DU, Price JB, *et al*. Arterial regeneration activity after prosthetic implantation. *Arch Surg* 1985; 120:315.

Guthrie CC. End-results of arterial restoration with devitalized tissue. *JAMA* 1919; 73:186.

Levin SM. Reminiscences and ruminations: Vascular surgery then and now. *Am J Surg* 1987; 154:158.

Smith RB III. Arthur B. Voorhees, Jr.: pioneer vascular surgeon. *J Vasc Surg* 1993; 18:341.

Smith RB III, Voorhees AB Jr., Davidson EA, *et al*. Toxic effects of ingested whole proteins and amino acid mixtures in patients with portal systemic hypertension. *Surg Forum* 1964; 15:98.

Voorhees AB Jr. Management of portal hypertension. *Bull NY Acad Med* 1959; 35:223.

Voorhees AB Jr. The development of arterial prostheses. A personal view. *Arch Surg* 1985; 120:289.

Voorhees AB Jr. The origin of the permeable arterial prosthesis: A personal reminiscence. *Surg Rounds* 1988; 11:79.

Voorhees AB Jr., Jaretzki A, Blakemore AH. The use of tubes constructed from vinyon "N" cloth in bridging arterial defects. A preliminary report. *Ann Surg* 1952; 135:332.

Voorhees AB Jr., Harris RC, Britton RC, *et al*. Portal hypertension in children: 98 cases. *Surgery* 1965; 58:540.

Voorhees AB Jr., Price JB Jr., Britton RC. Portasystemic shunting procedures for portal hypertension: twenty-six year experience in adults with cirrhosis of the liver. *Am J Surg* 1970; 119:501.

Voorhees AB Jr., Chaitman E, Schneider S, *et al*. Portal-systemic encephalopathy in the noncirrhotic patient: effect of portal-systemic shunting. *Arch Surg* 1973; 107:659.

# PART 5

# More divisions

# CHAPTER 12

# Contributions from the battlefield

*He who wishes to be a surgeon should go to war.*

*(Hippocrates)*

The archetypal military surgeon was the Greek physician, Claudius Galen, the "Clarissimus." Regarded as one of the greatest surgeons of antiquity, Galen studied at the school of philosophy in Pergamon, as well as the medical school. Galen became a surgeon to the gladiators in 158 AD and was so successful that he was reappointed to this prestigious position four additional times within 3 years (Figure 12.1).

Galen was best known for his treatment of wounds. He cared for fractures, dislocations, ruptured nerves and tendons, and a wide variety of penetrating injuries, with sutures and dressings. Galen utilized ligatures and relied heavily on cautery to control bleeding:

> The cautery is employed also in consumptives, patients with enlarged spleens, and habitual dislocation of the shoulder joint, in lacrymal fistula, in the resection of gangrenous tissue, where bleeding takes place on account of the opening of vessels, or in bleeding from other causes.

A thorough knowledge of anatomy and great technical skill allowed Galen to contribute to nearly all the surgical subspecialties including ophthalmology, genitourinary surgery, and neurosurgery. Galen's record was envied by the military surgeons who followed him, and he once attributed his successive reappointments as surgeon to the gladiators to his zero mortality rate.

During the 13 centuries following Galen's life, there was no shortage of wars or vascular injuries (Figure 12.2). The widely accepted method of treatment of hemorrhage continued to be boiling oil or the cautery. In 16th-century Europe, medicine retained strong ties to feudal customs and ancient dogma. Many physicians still referred to the works of Galen and his contemporaries in their treatment of patients. It required a renaissance to effect changes in wound care and to produce the next great military surgeon.

At about the time that Michelangelo was painting the Sistine Chapel, Ambroise Paré was born. He joined the French infantry at the age of 26. Paré's first campaign was the invasion of northern Italy, in the third war against Charles V, in 1536. Paré was insecure about his lack of experience and hesitated to apply boiling oil to gunshot wounds for fear of torturing his patients. Paré's fellow physicians reassured him, however, and he undertook this treatment. The Battle of Chateau de Villane was a particularly fierce one. So many injuries were sustained that the supply of heated oil was exhausted, and Paré was forced to use alternate means of caring for the wounded (Figure 12.3). A large measure of Paré's prominent position in the history of surgery is a result of that unex-

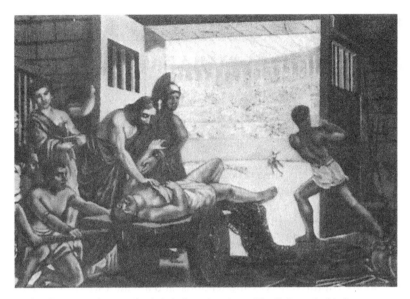

**Figure 12.1** Galen examines a wounded gladiator (courtesy of the Bettman Archive).

pected and seemingly unfortunate turn of events. His use of a simple dressing revolutionized the treatment of gunshot wounds and later encouraged him to test the ligature in the treatment of injured blood vessels. Paré described his discovery in the following way:

> I was at that time a fresh-water surgeon, since I had not yet seen treated wounds made by firearms. It is true I had read in Jean de Virgo, first book of *Wounds in General*, Chapter 8 that wounds made by firearms are poisoned because of the powder. For their cure he advised their cauterization with oil of elders mixed with a little theriac. Not to fail, this oil must be applied boiling, even though this would cause the wounded extreme pain. I wished to know first how to apply it, how the other Surgeons did their first dressings, which was to apply the oil as boiling as possible with the tents and setons. So I took heart to do as they did. Finally my oil was exhausted and I was forced to apply instead of a digestive made of egg yolk, rose oil and turpentine. That night I could not sleep easily, thinking that by failure of cauterizing, I would find the wounded in whom I had failed to put the oil, dead of poisoning. This made me get up early in the morning to visit them. There, beyond my hope, I found those on whom I had used the digestive medication feeling little pain in their wounds, without inflammation and swelling, having rested well through the night. The others on whom I had used the oil I found feverish, with great pain, swelling and inflammation around their wounds. Then I resolved never again to so cruelly burn the poor wounded by gunshot.

In 30 years as a military surgeon, Paré's skill and reputation soared (Figure 12.4). It was said that on the battlefield he was equivalent to 10 000 troops, for the soldiers knew his presence insured their greatest chance of survival. Armed with honesty and energy, Paré spent most of his career battling the medical dogmatism of his age. He elevated his profession to new heights, just as some of his contemporaries – such as Copernicus, Galileo, and Shakespeare – did theirs.

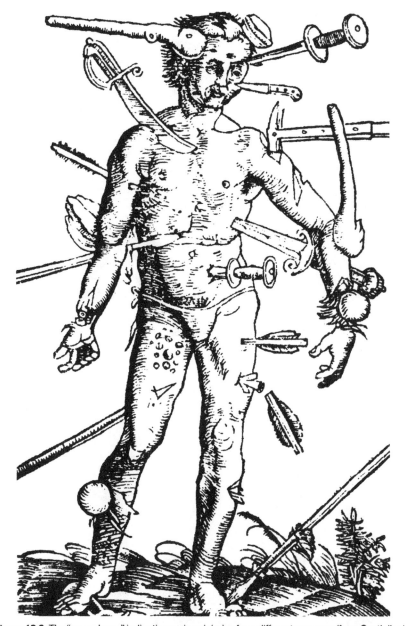

**Figure 12.2** The "wound man" indicating various injuries from different weapons (from Castiglioni A. *A History of Medicine*. New York: Alfred A. Knopf, 1947).

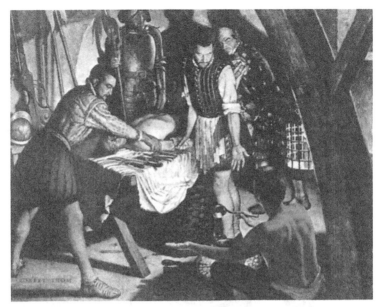

**Figure 12.3** *Ambroise Paré: Surgery Acquires Stature.* Paré exhausts his supply of boiling oil (from Parke, Davis & Co. *A History of Medicine in Pictures*, 1958).

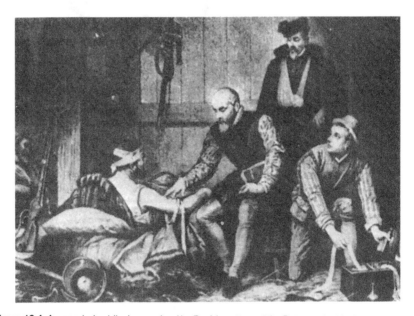

**Figure 12.4** A wounded soldier is examined by Paré (courtesy of the Bettman Archive).

The ligature as described by Paré would remain the treatment of choice for vascular injuries until 1952. Other well-known French military surgeons followed Paré, but none improved his methods. In 1718, Petit developed a screwed tourniquet to facilitate ligation of vessels during amputations. Fifty years later, Ravaton eschewed the cautery in favor of the ligature for control of bleeding, thereby reaffirming Pare's contributions.

Almost three centuries after Paré, another great wartime surgeon of France utilized the ligature for hemostasis. Dominique Jean Larrey was the foremost amputationist of the early 19th century and he put the ligature to frequent use (Figure 12.5). His greatest contribution, however, and one that is often overlooked, was the *ambulance volante*, or "flying ambulance" (Figure 12.6). This horse-drawn vehicle transported wounded soldiers from the battlefield to a rear treatment station where more thorough care could be administered.

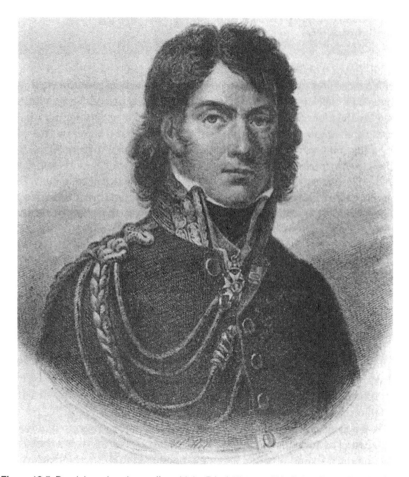

**Figure 12.5** Dominique Jean Larrey (from Major RA. *A History of Medicine*. Springfield, IL: Charles C Thomas, 1954).

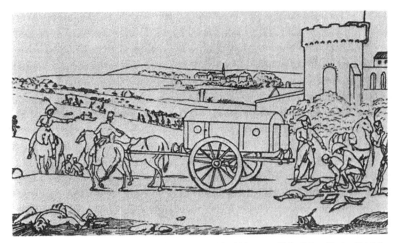

**Figure 12.6**  Larrey's "flying ambulance" (from Major RA. *A History of Medicine.* Springfield, IL: Charles C Thomas, 1954).

Larrey's concern for mobility and ready access to medical care for the injured foreshadowed the use of the helicopter more than 100 years later in southeast Asia, where the modern age of vascular surgery was conceived (Figure 12.7).

During the remainder of the 19th century, no further progress in the treatment of injured blood vessels was made. Even the foremost surgeon of this period, John Hunter, failed to speculate about the possibility of blood vessel repair. In one of his greatest works, *A Treatise on the Blood, Inflammation and Gun-Shot Wounds*, inspired by his experience as a military surgeon, no mention of this possibility was made. In fact, Hunter wrote of the ligature disparagingly, because it introduced a foreign body into the wound:

> The ligature used for tying a blood-vessel leaves an extraneous body in the wound; a part deprived of life by the instrument, etc. will become an extraneous substance, and the surfaces cannot always be brought into contact, so as to allow a perfect union to take place. In such cases, union is prevented by the blood losing in part its living principle, especially in those parts next to the external surface; and perhaps the art employed by the surgeon himself may insist in changing the original state of the wound, as the passing of needles and ligatures must always produce suppuration through the whole passage.

No large reports of treatment of acute arterial injuries appeared prior to World War I. This was because of poor record keeping and the inclusion by most reports of traumatic aneurysms and arterial–venous fistulas along with acute arterial injuries.

While it is generally accepted that the first widespread program of vascular repair in lieu of ligation took place during the Korean War, this is not the case. It was during the Balkan Wars that a lieutenant colonel in the Serbian Army Reserve initiated the first clinical program wherein injured blood vessels were managed preferentially by repair. The work of V. Soubbotitch remains obscure

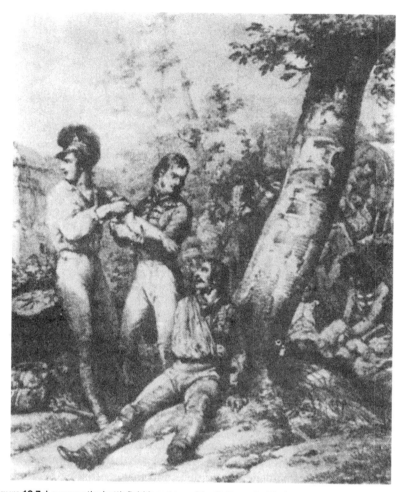

**Figure 12.7** Larrey on the battlefield (courtesy of the Bettman Archive).

despite its original publication in *The Lancet*. Soubbotitch presented his work from the Belgrade State Hospital to Rudolph Matas and others in London, in 1913 (Figure 12.8). In his management of 60 arterial and 17 venous injuries, 19 of the arteries and 13 veins were repaired by partial or circular suture. Soubbotitch eventually reported his results with 185 operations for vascular injuries in 1914. In describing repair of blood vessels Soubbotitch contended:

> Suture is certainly the most difficult and tedious proceeding, and is undoubtedly not the right treatment in all cases; nevertheless, it appears to be efficacious and to be indicated not only in those cases where it is absolutely necessary, but in others where it can be easily and aseptically carried out. . . . If it is possible to retain strips of the vessel, preserving its continuity, this may be done with advantage by putting the stitches into the wounds of the vessel wall in a transverse direction. In general an otherwise healthy vessel appears to stand dissection, if not too prolonged, by no means badly.

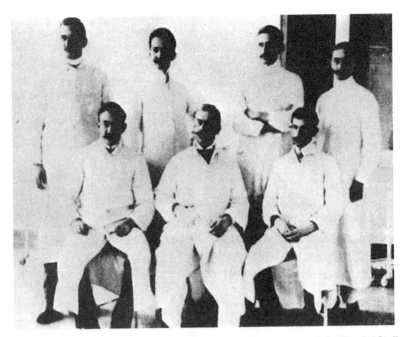

**Figure 12.8** V. Soubbotitch (front row, center) and members of his Belgrade State Hospital Staff. (From Rich NM, *et al*. The Matas/Soubbotitch connection. *Surgery* 1983; 937. Reprinted by permission from The C.V. Mosby Co.)

Four decades would elapse before similar attempts at vascular repair were undertaken during the Korean War.

Ligation remained the primary method of treating vascular injuries during World War I. The allied military surgeons believed that arterial repair could not be undertaken under battlefield conditions and that controlling hemorrhage alone would be sufficient. The largest account of vascular injuries in World War I was that of George Makins, England's Surgeon General. In his classic monograph *On Gunshot Injuries to the Blood Vessels*, he reviewed more than 1000 vascular injuries, yet failed to distinguish between acute and chronic wounds. In this and other reports, he clearly stated the preferred treatment of arterial injuries:

Little actual experience of the primary suture has been gained, but such as exists is not of a nature to encourage the hope of any great future for this method of treating wounded arteries in military surgery. I think it indubitable that in the present state of surgery direct ligation, when necessary, is likely to remain the only operation suitable for application to the primary injury, and this rule is still more applicable to the treatment of external recurrent or secondary haemorrhage.

In Makin's Hunterian Oration delivered before the Royal College of Surgeons in 1917, he did little more to promote the progress of vascular surgery with his comments on venous injuries:

Observation of a large number of coincident wounds of large arteries and veins has in no way endorsed the view that simultaneous occlusion of both artery and vein exercises any deleterious influence on the subsequent collateral arterial circulation and the vitality of the limb. . . . These considerations lead me not only to regard obligatory simultaneous occlusion of the main artery and vein as negligible factors in the risk of gangrene of a limb, but to hold, further, that the procedure is preferable whether the vein be wounded or not; the result of the combined procedure being to maintain within the limb for a longer period the smaller amount of blood supplied by the collateral arterial circulation, and hence to improve the conditions necessary for the preservation of the vitality of the limb.

Among the military surgeons representing the major disputants of World War I, only the Germans made a concerted effort to repair injured blood vessels. Several reports of successful vascular repairs appeared in their literature but were ignored. Jaeger attempted to use fresh arterial and venous homografts taken from limbs that had been severed on the battlefield, to replace wounded arteries. Most of these eventually thrombosed, however, and enthusiasm for Jaeger's innovative idea never developed.

Bertram Bernheim brought the United States close to considering a program of vascular repair when he traveled to France with much personal equipment and assistance to evaluate the efficacy of this treatment. In 2 years, however, he became so discouraged by the attempts of surgeons to repair injured blood vessels on the battlefield, that he abandoned the project, stating:

> Opportunities for carrying out the more modern procedures for the repair or reconstruction of damaged blood vessels were conspicuous by their absence during the recent military activities . . . . Not that blood vessels were immune from injury; not that gaping arteries and veins and vicariously united vessels did not cry out for relief by fine suture or anastomosis. They did, most eloquently, and in great numbers, but he would have been a foolhardy man who would have essayed sutures of arterial or venous trunks in the presence of such infections as were the rule in practically all of the battle wounded.

Despite the availability of whole blood, the recent discovery of antibiotics, more efficient evacuation of the wounded, and more accessible surgical treatment, World War II did little more than the first World War to advance vascular surgery beyond the thinking of Ambroise Paré. In their monumental treatise on battle injuries of the arteries in World War II, DeBakey (Figure 12.9) and Simeone reviewed 2471 cases of arterial wounds. Their meticulous analysis found only 81 instances of suture repair, resulting in an amputation rate of 36 percent; the rate following ligation was nearly 50 percent. Even though the results of suture repair compared favorably with those of ligation, and vein or prosthetic tube grafting, the authors cautioned that the successful cases comprised a "highly selective group of minimal wounds" and did not justify more widespread application of these techniques. The pessimism of DeBakey and Simeone regarding the possibility of repair of arterial battle injuries is apparent throughout their report:

> Therapeutic measures designed to save the limb are clearly applicable, at best, to not more than 20–25% of all such injuries, which should put to rest the overenthusiastic and even extravagant claims occasionally made as to the possibilities of salvage of limbs in battlewounds of the blood vessels. . . . From the preceding discussion, it is

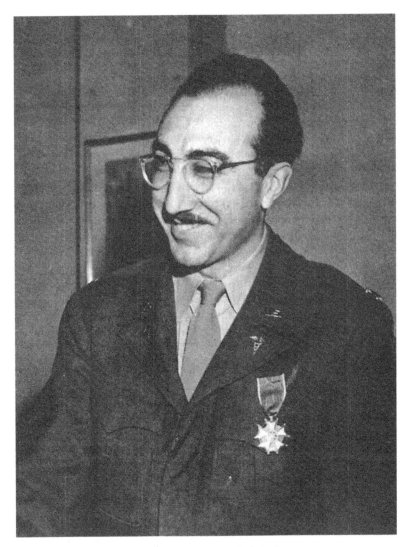

**Figure 12.9** Michael E. DeBakey (courtesy of Dr. Michael DeBakey).

clear that no procedure other than ligation is applicable to the majority of vascular injuries which come under the military surgeon's observation. It is not a procedure of choice. It is a procedure of stern necessity, for the basic purpose of controlling hemorrhage, as well as because of the location, type, size, and character of most battle injuries of the arteries.

Reflection upon these conclusions with hindsight might lead to harsh criticism of the authors, particularly in light of the great advances made during the Korean War a short time later. Examination of the exigencies of World War II reveals, however, that the recommendations of DeBakey and Simeone were based upon practical considerations. A major stumbling block for vascular repair during this war continued to be the inordinate delay between wounding and surgical treatment. In one sample of 58 cases of vascular injury, this time lag averaged 15.2 hours. Although efforts were made to bring surgical care as close to the front lines as possible in World War II, it was deemed unfeasible to attempt definitive care of wounded vessels at the battalion aid station level. With such long delays before treatment of most of these injuries, attempts at revascularization would have been fruitless. A critical reduction in this delay was essential, and a combination of events would make this possible during the upcoming conflict in Korea.

A second obstacle to effective vascular repair in World War II was infection. The importance of radical debridement of all contaminated wounds, as well as the role of antibiotics and fluid resuscitation, had not yet been fully appreciated. Widespread institution of each of these important practices contributed to the forthcoming success on the battlefields of southeast Asia.

DeBakey and Simeone recognized the possibility of vascular repair under more favorable conditions when they wrote:

> All battle wounds are potentially infected, it is true, but if adequate debridement can be done, surgical procedures directed toward the treatment of the vascular injury can be done at the same time with a high degree of safety. It is not infection, but the other circumstances just outlined, which now prevent reparative procedures in most battle injuries of the blood vessels.

One additional important contribution of this report was the repudiation of Makin's earlier advice to ligate veins adjacent to arterial injuries. DeBakey and Simeone pointed to the complete lack of physiologic data to support such a practice, and concluded that it should be abandoned. They also noted that Matas had recognized this 25 years earlier when he observed: "The danger of peripheral gangrene is always made doubly worse by the simultaneous injury of the accompanying or satellite vein."

In partial recognition of the unwillingness of DeBakey and Simeone to rule out the possibility of vascular repair in wartime, a program was instituted at the Walter Reed Army Hospital in 1949 to study blood vessel repair and replacement with fresh and preserved venous and arterial homografts. Realizing the importance of reducing the time delay between vascular injury and treatment, Hughes, Jahnke, Seeley, and their colleagues also attempted to determine the maximum time between blood supply to an extremity and muscle cell death.

Soon after the inception of this study, the Korean War began. The Walter Reed Army Hospital was designated as the vascular specialty center, and within a short period several hundred patients with traumatic aneurysms, arterial–venous fistulas, and ligated major vessels were referred. The early treatment of these lesions followed the guidelines established during World War II and consisted of simple ligation. Continued evaluation of these patients, however, revealed the unacceptable high rate of arterial insufficiency that ensued. A new policy of maintenance or restoration of vascular continuity was begun in 1952. With the exception of the aforementioned work by Soubbotitch, this represented the first deviation from the practice initiated by Paré 400 years earlier. Utilizing direct anastomosis, lateral repair, and graft replacement, the first 98 patients were operated upon with a 96 percent initial success rate.

Encouraged by these results, a contingent of the Army Surgical Research Team, consisting of Hughes, Jenke, Howard, and Artz, departed for southeast Asia. With newly available vascular instruments, antibiotics, blood products, and the military's newest *ambulance volante*, the helicopter, vascular repair was begun in the mobile army surgical hospitals (MASH) (Figure 12.10). The first 130 cases were performed with an 89 percent limb salvage rate. A new era in vascular surgery was born. Most repairs were accomplished by direct anastomosis or vein graft insertion. Working at the same time in the

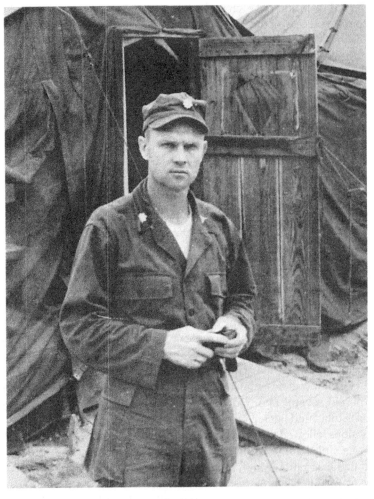

**Figure 12.10** Carl W. Hughes, 8055 MASH unit, Korea, 1953 (courtesy of Dr. Norman Rich).

First Marine Corps division, Spencer performed similar procedures utilizing arterial homografts.

In 1952, Richard Warren visited Korea as a consultant to the Surgeon General and discussed the feasibility of vascular repair with surgeons in the field. Following his report, vascular instruments and sutures were distributed to all MASH units. In addition, the principles and techniques of repair of acute vascular injuries were demonstrated to military surgeons throughout Korea by members of the Surgical Research Team. Ligation of major arteries during World War II had resulted in a 49 percent amputation rate. In his overall analysis of 304 major arterial repairs during the Korean War, Hughes eventually reported a 13 percent amputation rate. Repair of the injured blood vessel had become an accepted practice.

The battlefield furnishes the best opportunity to treat large numbers of any type of injury in a brief period of time. The outbreak of fighting in Vietnam provided the chance to advance the lessons learned in Korea, as well as to study anew the repair of injured blood vessels. Under the direction of Rich and Hughes, the Vietnam Vascular Registry was begun in 1966 to document and analyze all vascular injuries treated in army hospitals in Vietnam (Figure 12.11). In a review of 1000 acute arterial injuries from this war, managed primarily by vein grafting or end-to-end anastomosis, a limb salvage rate of 87 percent was achieved. Although these results appear similar to those obtained in Korea, they actually reflect further improvements in transportation of the wounded and in vascular surgical techniques. More efficient evacuation of the wounded in Vietnam allowed patients who would not have survived in Korea to reach surgical aid. Many surgeons with varying degrees of skill and training undertook vascular repairs in Vietnam, compared with the few with a special interest in the field in Korea. Finally, as indicated by Rich, the new-found enthusiasm for salvaging threatened extremities led to more frequent heroic attempts when primary amputation was indicated. A variety of additional contributions to vascular surgery have emerged from the Vietnam Vascular Registry. These include studies of complications from arterial repair, management of venous injuries, missile emboli, and concomitant fractures and vascular injuries. The knowledge gained through this unique registry has greatly facilitated the civilian practice of every present-day vascular surgeon.

At the end of the 20th century, civil wars in the Middle East and the former Yugoslavia provided additional experience with the treatment of vascular injuries. In 1995, Sfeir reported the results of 16 years of vascular trauma treatment at the American University of Beirut Medical Center. The report included 386 patients with 118 popliteal, 252 femoral, and 16 tibial arterial injuries. The mortality rate was 2.3 percent, all resulting from femoral artery injuries. The limb salvage rate was 94 percent and it was noted that delay in repair (more than 6 hours), associated femoral fractures, and shock on admission led to an increased amputation rate.

More recently Davidović reported the early postoperative results of 44 patients with popliteal artery injuries treated with bypass grafts, during the civil

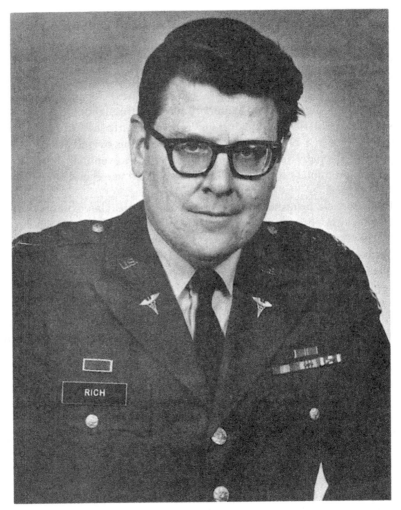

**Figure 12.11** Norman M. Rich (courtesy of Dr. Norman Rich).

war in Yugoslavia. The graft patency rate was 100 percent and the limb salvage rate was 28 percent. Factors contributing to limb loss included concomitant bone fractures, secondary reconstructions, secondary hemorrhage from an infected graft, and wounds resulting from an explosion rather than a gunshot.

In 1997, Radonić reported the results of 67 patients with femoral vein or artery injuries. There were a total of 70 arterial and 49 venous injuries. Autogenous repairs or ligation were used in all cases, and a remarkable 97 percent survival was achieved. The 95 percent limb salvage rate supported the immediate and coordinated approach of the Split Clinic Hospital to femoral vascular trauma.

In 2000, Velinovic summarized the Clinical Center of Serbia experience with 106 arterial injuries in 97 patients. They achieved a limb salvage rate of 78 percent and also found that associated injuries, and the need for secondary operations, led to a higher amputation rate.

## Bibliography

Bernheim B. Blood vessel surgery in the war. *Surg Gynecol Obstet* 1920; 30:564.

Davidović L, Lotina S, Kostic D, *et al*. Popliteal artery war injuries. *Cardiovasc Surg* 1997; 5:37.

DeBakey ME, Simeone FA. Battle injuries of the arteries in World War II. An analysis of 2,471 cases. *Ann Surg* 1946; 123:534.

Degenshein GA. Golden age of surgery. *Surg Clin N Am* 1978; 58:930.

Haberland HFO. Zur technik der gefaesschirurgie. *Beitrage Zur Klin Chirurg* 1916; 100:52.

Hamby WB. *The Case Reports and Autopsy Records of Ambroise Paré*. Springfield: Charles C. Thomas, 1960.

Hughes CW. Arterial repair during the Korean War. *Am Surg* 1958; 147:555.

Hughes CW. Vascular surgery in the armed forces. *Milit Med* 1959; 124:30.

Hughes CW, Jahnke EJ Jr. A five-year follow-up study of 215 lesions. The surgery of traumatic arteriovenous fistulas and aneurysms. *Ann Surg* 1958; 148:790.

Hunter J. *A Treatise on the Blood, Inflammation and Gun-Shot Wounds. 1794.* Birmingham: Gryphon Editions, Ltd, 1982.

Jaeger E. Zur technik der blutgefaessenaht. *Beitr Klin Chir* 1915; 97:553.

Kuttner H. Neue erfahrungen in der kriegschirurgie der grossen blut-gefaesstamme. *Berl Klin Wschr* 1916; 53:132.

Makins GH. Gunshot injuries of arteries. *Br Med J* 1913; 2:1569.

Makins GH. The Hunterian Oration on the influence exerted by the military experience of John Hunter on himself and the military surgeon of to-day. *Lancet* 1917; 1:249.

Makins GH. *On Gunshot Injuries to the Blood Vessels*. Bristol: John Wright & Sons, Ltd, 1919.

Matas R. Surgery of the vascular system. In: Keen WW, ed. *Surgery: Its Principles and Practice, by Various Authors*. Philadelphia: WB Saunders Co, 1921.

Radonić V, Baric D, Giuniot L, *et al*. War injuries of the femoral artery and vein: a report on 67 cases. *Cardiovasc Surg* 1998; 5:641.

Rich NM, Hughes CW. Vietnam vascular registry: A preliminary report. *Surgery* 1969; 65:218.

Rich NM, Hughes CW. Fifty years' progress in vascular injuries. *Bull Am Coll Surg* June, 1972.

Rich NM, Baugh JH, Hughes CW. Acute arterial injuries in Vietnam: 1,000 cases. *J Trauma* 1970; 10:359.

Rich NM, Hughes CW, Baugh JH. Management of venous injuries. *Ann Surg* 1970; 171:724.

Rich NM, Baugh JH, Hughes CW. Significance of complications associated with vascular repairs performed in Vietnam. *Arch Surg* 1970; 100:646.

Rich NM, Metz CW Jr., Hutton JE Jr., *et al*. Internal vs external fixation of fractures with concomitant vascular injuries in Vietnam. *J Trauma* 1971; 11:463.

Rich NM, Hobson RW, Fedde CW, et al. Acute common femoral arterial trauma. *J Trauma* 1975; 15:628.

Rich NM, Collins GJ Jr., Anderson CA, *et al*. Missile emboli. *J Trauma* 1978; 18:236.

Seeley SF, Hughes CW, Jahnke EJ Jr. Direct anastomosis versus ligation and excision in traumatic arteriovenous fistulas and aneurysms. *Surg Forum, Clin Cong Am Coll Surg*. Philadelphia: WB Saunders Co, 1953.

Sfeir RE, Khoury GS, Kenaan MK. Vascular trauma to the lower extremity: the Lebanese war experience. *Cardiovasc Surg* 1995; 3:653.

Soubbotitch V. Military experiences of traumatic aneurysms. *Lancet* 1913; 2:720.

Soubbotitch V. Experience in wartime surgical treatment of traumatic aneurysms (Serbo-Croatian). *Serb Med Soc* 1914; 20:1.

Spencer FC, Grewe RV. The management of arterial injuries in battle casualties. *Ann Surg* 1955; 141:304.

Toledo-Pereyra LH. Galen's contribution to surgery. *J Hist Med* 1973; 10:357.

Toledo-Pereyra LH. A surgeon of antiquity. *Surg Gynecol Obstet* 1974; 138:767.

Velinovic MM, Davidovic BL, Lotina IS, *et al.* Complications of operative treatment of injuries of peripheral arteries. *Cardiovasc Surg* 2000; 8:256.

Von Haberer H. Diagnose und die behandlung der gefaessverletzungen. *Munch Med Wschr* 1918; 1:363.

Wangensteen OH, Wangensteen SD, Klinger CF. Wound management of Ambroise Paré and Dominique Larrey, great French military surgeons of the 16th and 19th centuries. *Bull Hist Med* 1972; 46:207.

Warren R. *Report to the Surgeon General, Dept of the Army*. Washington, DC, April, 1952.

# CHAPTER 13

# Venous surgery

*The legges . . . whey they are offended or wounded are very perilous, because unto them runneth a great quantity of humors . . . [edematous ulcers] are troublesome and curious to heale.*

*(Thomas Vicary)*

The great Indian surgeon of antiquity, Sushruta, offered the first recorded description of varicose veins (Figure 13.1). In the second volume of his *Samhit*, he discussed *siragranthi* or "aneurysms of the veins." He asserted that "straining or exertion by pressure" caused varicosities to develop, and that they were incurable. In addition, Sushruta described thrombophlebitis as a related condition, also difficult to treat, which was "shifting and slightly painful."

Several centuries later, Hippocrates demonstrated a basic understanding of the pathophysiology of venous insufficiency (Figure 13.2). He taught that standing should be discouraged in patients with lower extremity ulcers. Varicosities represented "an influx of blood into the veins" and Hippocrates further cautioned against attempts to excise these lesions since large ulcers would result. He recommended the use of compression bandages to treat them. Curious curative properties were ascribed to varicose veins by Hippocrates in several of his aphorisms: "If varicose veins or hemorrhoids occur during mania, the mania is cured."

Many middle-aged men of today might find some encouragement in another Hippocratic pronouncement: "The bald are not subject to varicose veins; but should they occur, the hairs are reproduced."

In the first century AD, Celsus used linen bandages and various types of plaster to treat leg ulcers. A century later, Galen elaborated a description of the surgical treatment of varicose veins, which might suffice for the purposes of a textbook today:

In varicose veins of the legs we mark out the whole extent of them by scratches on the outside, then put them on their backs, take hold of the skin surface, and divide that first, then lift up the varicosity with a hook and tie it off, and do the same thing at all the incisions. Or we pull them out with a varicocele hook and cut off the ends, or we pass thread through the coil of the veins with a probe and pull them up and take them out.

During the ensuing 16 centuries, Galen's humoral dynamics, with the notion of the to-and-fro motion of blood and its spirits, was the basis for the prevailing theory of the etiology of varicose veins. Varices were thought to be a repository for deleterious humors and were safe unless pressed back into the circulation.

In 1579, Ambroise Paré wrote of the treatment of varicose veins:

It is best not to meddle with such as are inveterate; for of such being cured there is to be feared a reflux of the melancholy bloud to the noble parts, whence there may be imminent danger of malign ulcers, a cancer, madness or suffocation.

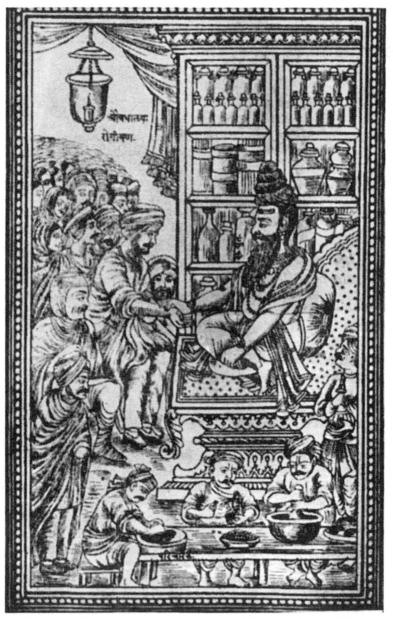

**Figure 13.1** The teaching of medicine by Sushruta: from an 18th-century Indian print (from Castiglioni A. *A History of Medicine*. New York: Alfred A. Knopf, 1947).

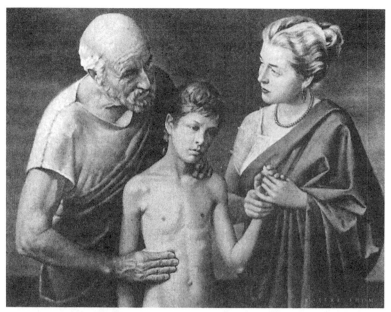

**Figure 13.2** *Hippocrates: Medicine Becomes a Science* (from Parke, Davis & Co. *A History of Medicine in Pictures*, 1958).

Until the end of the 19th century, the most effective therapy for all forms of venous disease, despite Galen's theory, and unchanged since Hippocrates's exegesis, remained elevation and compression. In 1868, John Gay, a London surgeon, wrote that the popular term "varicose ulcer" was misleading and recommended changing it to "venous ulcer" (Figure 13.3). He reasoned that, since these ulcers were not invariably associated with visible varicose veins, other abnormalities of the deep or communicating venous system might be implicated in their cause.

In 1896, the first improvement in compression therapy since Hippocrates was developed by the German dermatologist Unna. He introduced his plaster boot as a new form of medical therapy, and it remains in wide use today.

Like many developments in vascular surgery, the roots of the present era of venous reconstruction are discovered in the work of Carrel and Guthrie. As early as 1906, they experimented with grafts placed into the venous system.

In 1916, 10 years after the work of Carrel and Guthrie, John Homans expanded upon the theories of Gay by offering a classification of venous disorders (Figure 13.4). Venous surgery up to this time consisted of saphenous venous ligation, popularized by Trendelenburg; ligation of superficial varicosities, or excision of the entire saphenous vein (Figure 13.5). Homans suggested that operative treatment of varicose veins and ulcers should be based upon the specific abnormality causing them. As an example he wrote:

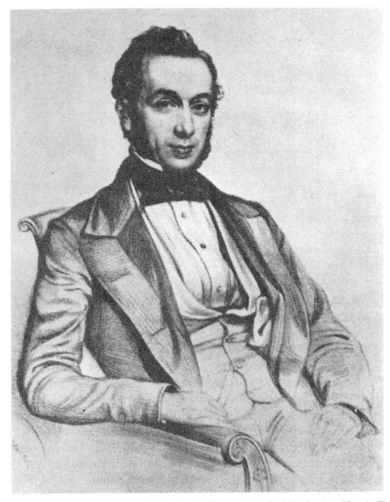

**Figure 13.3** John Gay (from Anning ST. The historical aspects. In: Dodd H, Cockett FB, eds. *The Pathology and Surgery of the Veins of the Lower Limb*. London: Churchill-Livingstone, 1976).

Surface varix complicated by varicosity of the perforating veins requires for its cure not only eradication of the great saphenous vein, but a thorough exploration of the lower leg in order to ligate varicose perforating veins.

The first use of phlebography by Beberich and Hirsch in 1923 was a milestone in the diagnosis of venous disorders. The first attempt to quantify the degree of venous insufficiency was made by Barber in 1925. His "blood manometer" consisted of a long glass tube, rubber tubing, and an 18-gauge needle which were used to obtain direct measurements of lower extremity venous pressure.

Important surgical landmarks of this decade included the first venous thrombectomy by Bazy, performed for a case of effort thrombosis of the axillary

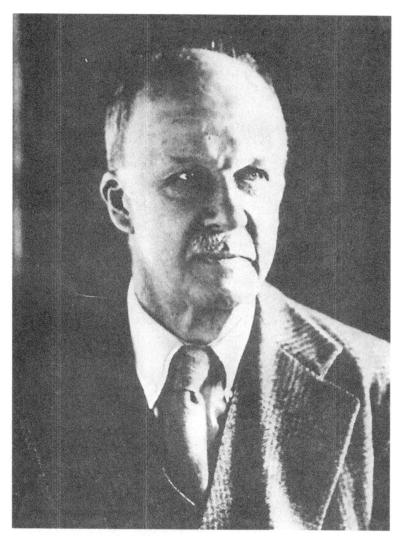

**Figure 13.4** John Homans (courtesy of Dr. R. Clement Darling).

vein. In 1938, Laewen described important considerations for the maintenance of venous patency following thrombectomy.

A major contribution to the understanding of venous diseases and the specific role of the communicating veins was a report by Linton in 1938 (Figure 13.6). He described the specific anatomy of these veins and the operative approaches to them. Based on data from 50 "flap" operations and additional cadaver dissections, Linton divided the communicating veins into three main groups and described their surgical exposure, thereby forming the basis for the Linton procedure. Linton pursued his study of venous abnormalities and made

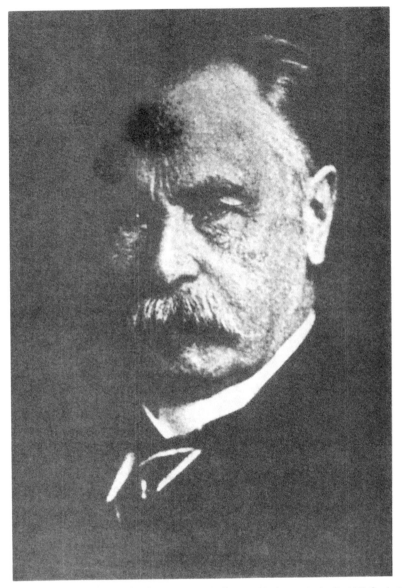

**Figure 13.5** Friedrich Trendelenburg (from Anning ST. The historical aspects. In: Dodd H, Cockett FB, eds. *The Pathology and Surgery of the Veins of the Lower Limb*. London: Churchill-Livingstone, 1976).

many more contributions to the management of venous diseases. He summarized the state of venous surgery before the first meeting of the North American chapter of the International Society of Angiology in 1952:

> The interruption of the deep venous system prevents a direct reflux flow of blood down these large veins and at the same time favors redirecting the returning blood

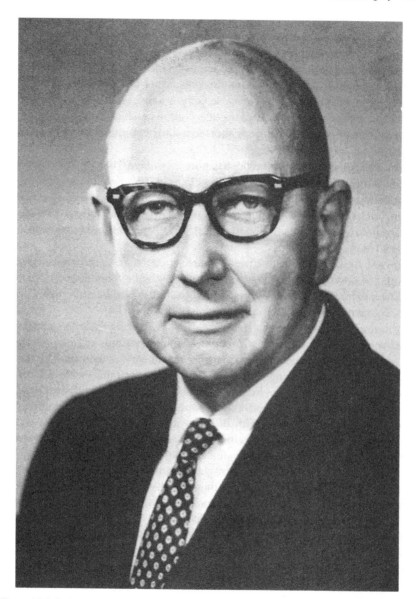

**Figure 13.6** Robert Linton (courtesy of Dr. R. Clement Darling).

through smaller venous channels that may have competent valves. Resection of the
deep fascia favors a reduction in the lymphedema. The general effects of these various
steps, it is believed, although the ambulatory venous pressure of the limb may not be
reduced, is to restore in part the function of the venous heart. This effect is further
enhanced by the wearing of a heavy weight, two way stretch elastic stocking. The
results of this method of treatment have been extremely encouraging during the past

five years, but further observation will be necessary to determine if they will continue to justify such an extensive surgical procedure.

The hypothesis originally proffered by Gay and Homans, that abnormalities other than varicose veins gave rise to venous insufficiency, was eventually confirmed by Gunnar Bauer of Sweden. In 1948, Bauer utilized descending phlebography in 100 patients with varicose veins and leg ulcers, to demonstrate a high incidence of abnormalities of the deep venous system. Bauer also reported favorable results with resection of a short segment of popliteal vein in 54 of these patients.

The present era of venous reconstruction, coeval with the advent of modern arterial surgical techniques, began in the 1950s. In 1952, Kunlin used a segment of saphenous vein to bypass an obstructed external iliac vein; the graft remained patent for 3 weeks. One year later, Warren reported transplantation of the saphenous vein to a deeper position in the thigh, for postphlebitic syndrome in a 48-year-old man.

In 1957, Eduardo Palma of Uruguay performed the first saphenous–femoral venous crossover graft in a 35-year-old female who had developed refractory left lower extremity venous ulcers following a cholecystectomy (Figure 13.7). In 1960, Palma reported seven additional uses of this operation.

Although progress in arterial surgery was rapid during the 1950s and 1960s, improvements in venous reconstruction were slow in coming. Venous surgery had garnered less interest than arterial surgery for several reasons. The results obtained from arterial surgery were usually more dramatic, since the consequences of venous disorders may be tolerated for years. The different types of venous abnormalities rendered the pathophysiology of venous insufficiency more complex, often resulting in difficulty identifying which patient would benefit most. A simple bypass, as in the arterial circuit, was rarely all that was needed. Finally, venous reconstructions were frequently more difficult than arterial, as veins are collapsible, thin-walled tubes with fine valves in a low-pressure system. Graft patency and the integrity of specific reparative techniques were therefore more difficult to maintain. All of these factors suppressed interest and progress in venous reconstruction.

Early experimental attempts at venous grafting and bypass were performed by Dale and Scott, Steinman, Moore and Young, and others during the 1960s. In 1967, Husni adapted the *in situ* vein bypass technique to treat incompetence of the femoral and popliteal veins. In 1970, he presented a series of 20 patients so treated, with success in 16.

In 1968, Psathakis described his "substitute valve" at the popliteal vein level using a length of gracilis tendon (Figure 13.8). This eventually led to the efforts of Taheri and others, beginning in 1980, to transplant normal valve-bearing venous segments into diseased areas.

Although it had long been recognized that incompetent femoral vein valves could also produce venous insufficiency, direct repair of these structures was not attempted until 1968, when Kistner reported his first case. In 1975 he presented his experience with femoral vein valve repair in 14 patients and 17 lower

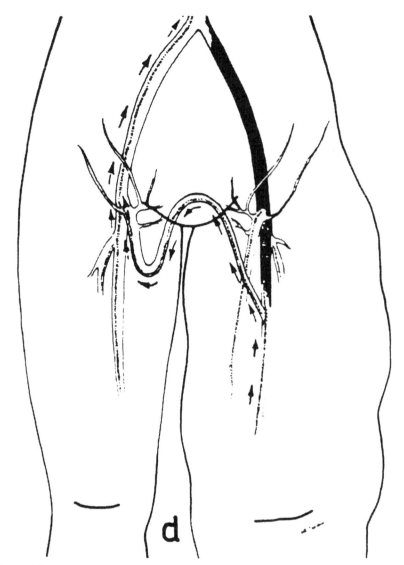

**Figure 13.7** The saphenous–femoral venous crossover graft of Palma (from Palma E, Esperon R. Vein transplants and grafts in the surgical treatment of postphlebitic syndrome. *J Cardiovasc Surg* 1960; 1:94).

extremities before the International Society of Cardiovascular Surgery. The long-term results were excellent (Figure 13.9).

It was only a matter of time before prosthetic grafts made their way into the venous system. In 1979, Rosenthal used a prosthetic interposition graft for a case of portal hypertension. Thirteen years later, Gloviczki reported his results with three PTFE grafts used for reconstruction of the superior vena cava. Two

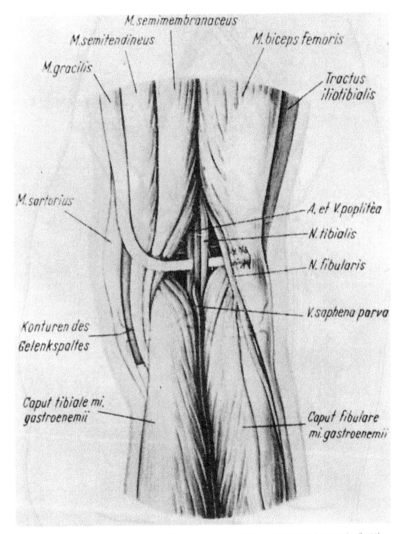

**Figure 13.8** Psathakis' "substitute valve" (from Psathakis N. Has the "substitute valve" at the popliteal vein solved the problem of venous insufficiency of the lower extremity? *J Cardiovasc Surg* 1968; 9:64).

required early thrombectomy, and two were patent after 2 and 5 years respectively. The median patency rate of eleven inferior vena cava PTFE grafts was 9 months and an atrial–caval Dacron graft remained patent for 3 years. In 1997, Alimi also reported favorable results with prosthetic reconstruction of iliac veins.

In recognition of the different etiologies and locations of lower extremity venous disease, the CEAP classification was devised in 1994. Under the auspices of the American Venous Forum, this classification defined the clinical class

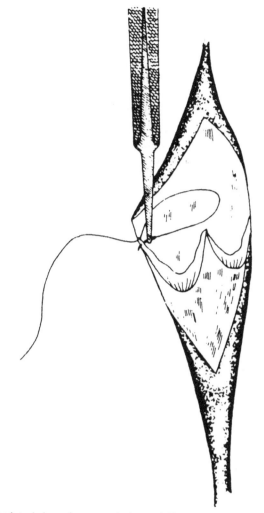

**Figure 13.9** Kistner's technique of venous valvular repair (from Kistner R. Surgical repair of a venous valve. *Straub Clin Proc* 1968; 34:41).

(C), the etiology (E), the anatomic (A) distribution, and the pathologic (P) mechanism of the venous disease. Seven classes were designated according to the clinical signs, and severity and disability rating scales were also devised.

In 1996, Gloviczki reported preliminary results with endoscopic subfacial division of perforating veins. A mean of 4.4 veins were divided in each of 11 extremities, and ulcer improvement or healing was noted in 10. In 1999, the North American Subfacial Endoscopic Perforator Surgery Registry reported results with 146 patients followed for a mean of 2 years. Perforator interruption combined with superficial reflux ablation was effective in healing ulcers. In patients with post-thrombotic limbs, however, recurrent or new ulcer development remained a problem.

Most venous disorders are treated without surgery, and the mainstay of treatment was developed by an engineer, not a surgeon. Conrad Jobst designed brush-making machines and eventually obtained more than 40 patents. Jobst suffered from varicose veins for most of his life, and began the first of many sclerotherapy sessions at the Henry Ford Hospital in 1930. He eventually recognized that venous insufficiency resulted from excessive hydrostatic pressure, and designed the first ambulatory gradient compression stockings for the treatment of venous insufficiency. Half a century later, Jobst's innovation remains the most important therapy for this disorder.

The first use of intravenous sclerotherapy was reported by Pravaz in 1840; he used absolute alcohol and eventually resorted to ferric chloride.

In 1910, Scharf reported his results with injection of sublimate into his own varicose veins, and into the veins of 90 patients. In 1916, Linser recommended perchloride of mercury and ambulatory treatments. In the first half of the 20th century, many other substances were used for sclerotherapy including grape sugar and sodium citrate; they were all abandoned, however, owing to allergic reactions, skin sloughing, pain, and death in several cases.

In 1939, McAusland reported his successful treatment with sclerotherapy of 10 000 patients. He advocated injection into empty veins, postsclerotherapy compression, and minimal concentrations of sodium morrhuate to limit complications. Two years later, Brunstein reiterated the value of McAusland's techniques, and sclerotherapy became an accepted treatment for venous insufficiency.

## Bibliography

AbuRahma AF, Robinson PA, Boland JP. Clinical hemodynamic and anatomic predictors of long-term outcome of lower extremity veno-venous bypasses. *J Vasc Surg* 1991; 14: 635.

Alimi YS, DiMauro P, Fabre D, Juhan C. Iliac vein reconstructions to treat acute and chronic venous occlusive disease. *J Vasc Surg* 1997; 25:673.

Anning ST. The historical aspects. In: Dodd H, Cockett FB, eds. *The Pathology and Surgery of the Veins of the Lower Limb*. London: Churchill, Livingstone, 1976.

Barber RF, Shatara FI. The varicose disease. *NY State Med J* 1925; 25:162.

Bauer G. The etiology of leg ulcers and their treatment by resection of the popliteal vein. *J Int Chir* 1948; 8:937.

Bazy L. Thrombose de la veine axillaire droite (thrombophlebite dite "par effort"). Phlébotomie ablation des caillots. Suture de la veine. *Bull Soc Nation Chir* (Paris) 1926; 52:529.

Beberich J, Hirsch S. Die roentgenologische darstellung der arterien und venen in lebenden menschen. *Klin Wschr* 1923; 49:222b.

Bhishagratna KL. *An English Translation of the Sushruta Samhita*. Varanasi: Chowkhamba Sanskrit Series Office, 1963.

Brunstein IA. Prevention of discomfort and disability in the treatment of varicose veins. *Am J Surg* 1941; 54:362.

Carrel A, Guthrie CC. Uniterminal and biterminal venous transplantation. *Surg Gynecol Obstet* 1906; 2:266.

Cerino M, McGraw JY, Luke JC. Autogenous vein graft replacement of thrombosed deep veins. Experimental approach to the treatment of the postphlebitic syndrome. *Surgery* 1964; 55: 123.

Clowes W. Extra-anatomical bypass of iliac vein obstruction: Use of a synthetic (expanded polytetrafluoroethylene [Goretex] graft). *Arch Surg* 1980; 115:767.

Coar T. *The Aphorisms of Hippocrates with a Translation into Latin and English. 1822.* Birmingham: Gryphon Editions, Ltd, 1982.

Dale WA, Scott HW Jr. Grafts of the venous system. *Surgery* 1963; 53:52.

Dale WA, Harris J, Terry RB. Polytetrafluoroethylene reconstruction of the inferior vena cava. *Surgery* 1984; 95:625.

Dos Santos JC. La phlebographic direct. *J Int Chir* 1938; 3:625.

Fiore AC, Cromartie RS, Peigh PS, et al. Prosthetic replacement for the thoracic vena cava. *J Thorac Cardiovasc Surg* 1982; 84:560.

Gay J. On varicose disease of the lower extremities. *The Lettsomian Lectures of 1867.* London: Churchill, 1868.

Gloviczki P, Pairolero PC, Toomey BJ, *et al.* Reconstruction of large veins for nonmalignant venous occlusive disease. *J Vasc Surg* 1992; 16:750.

Gloviczki P, Cambria RA, Rhee RY, *et al.* Surgical technique and preliminary results of endoscopic subfascial division of perforating veins. *J Vasc Surg* 1996; 23:517.

Gloviczki P, Bergan JJ, Rhodes JM, *et al.* North American Study Group: mid-term results of endoscopic perforator vein interruption for chronic venous insufficiency: lessons learned from the North American Subfascial Endoscopic Perforator Surgery (NASEPS) registry. *J Vasc Surg* 1999; 29:489.

Homans J. The operative treatment of varicose veins and ulcers, based upon a classification of these lesions. *Surg Gynecol Obstet* 1916; 22:143.

Homans J. The etiology and treatment of varicose ulcer of the leg. *Surg Gynecol Obstet* 1917; 24:300.

Howard-Jones N. A critical study of the origins and early development of hypodermic medication. *J Hist Med* 1947; 2:201.

Husni EA. In situ saphenopopliteal bypass graft for incompetence of the femoral and popliteal veins. *Surg Gynecol Obstet* 1970; 2:279.

Ijima H, Sakurai J, Mori M, et al. Temporary arteriovenous fistula for venous reconstruction using a synthetic graft: Clinical and experimental evaluation. *J Cardiovasc Surg* 1981; 222: 480.

Kistner R. Surgical repair of a venous valve. *Straub Clin Proc* 1968; 34:41.

Kistner R. Surgical repair of the incompetent femoral vein valve. *Arch Surg* 1975; 110:1336.

Kunlin J. The reestablishment of venous circulation with grafts in cases of obliteration from trauma or thrombophlebitis. *Mem Acad Clin* 1953; 79:109.

Laewen A. Weitere erfahrungen ueber operative thrombenentfernung bei venenthrombose. *Arch Klin Chir* 1938; 193:723.

Linser F. Uber die Konservative Behandlung der Varicen. *Med Klin* 1916; 12:897.

Linton RR. The communicating veins of the lower leg and the operative technic for their ligation. *Ann Surg* 1938; 107:582.

Linton RR. Modern concepts in the treatment of the postphlebitic syndrome with ulcerations of the lower extremity. *Angiology* 1952; 3:431.

Linton RR, Harry IB Jr. Postthrombotic syndrome of the lower extremity. *Surgery* 1948; 24:452.

Linton RR, Keeley JK. The postphlebitic varicose ulcer. *Am Heart J* 1939; 17:27.

McAusland S. The modern treatment of varicose veins. *Med Press* 1939; 201:404.

Moore TC, Young NK. Experimental replacement and bypass of large veins. *Bull Soc Int Chir* 1964; 23:274.

O'Donnell TF, Fredricks R. Venous obstruction: an analysis of one hundred thirty-seven cases with hemodynamic, venographic, and clinical correlations. *J Vasc Surg* 1991; 14:305.

O'Donnell TF, Mackey WC, Shepard AD, Callow AD. Clinical hemodynamic and anatomic follow-up of direct venous reconstruction. *Arch Surg* 1987; 122:474.

Palma E, Esperon R. Vein transplants and grafts in the surgical treatment of postphlebitic syndrome. *J Cardiovasc Surg* 1960; 1:94.

Psathakis N. Has the "substitute valve" at the popliteal vein solved the problem of venous insufficiency of the lower extremity? *J Cardiovasc Surg* 1968; 9:64.

Raju S. Venous insufficiency of the lower limb and stasis ulceration. Changing concepts and management. *Ann Surg* 1983; 197:688.

Rhodes JM, Gloviczki P, Canton LG, *et al*. Factors affecting clinical outcome following endoscopic perforator vein ablation. *Am J Surg* 1998; 176:162.

Rhodes JM, Gloviczki P, Canton LG, *et al*. Endoscopic perforator vein division with ablation of superficial reflux improves venous hemodynamics. *J Vasc Surg* 1998; 28:839.

Rogoff SM, DeWeese JA. Phlebography of the lower extremity. *JAMA* 1960; 172:1599.

Rosenthal D, Deterling RA, O'Donnell TF, et al. Interposition grafting with expanded polytetrafluoroethylene for portal hypertension. *Surg Gynecol Obstet* 1979; 148:378.

Scharf P. Ein neues Verfahren der intravenosen Behandlung der Varicositaten der Unterextremitaten. *Berliner Klin Wochenschr* 1910; 13:582.

Smirk FM. Observations on the causes of oedema in congestive heart failure. *Clin Sci* 1936; 2:317.

Steinman C, Alpert J, Haimovici H. Inferior vena cava bypass grafts: An experimental evaluation of a temporary arteriovenous fistula on their long-term patency. *Arch Surg* 1966; 93:747.

Taheri SA, Lazar L, Elias S, *et al*. Surgical treatment of postphlebitic syndrome with vein valve transplant. *Am J Surg* 1982; 144:221.

Toledo-Pereyra LH. Galen's contribution to surgery. *J Hist Med* 1973; Oct, 357.

Trendelenburg F. Ueber die unterbindung der vena saphena magna bei unterschenkelvaricen. *Beit Klin Chir* 1890; 7:195.

Unna PG. Ueber paraplaste: Eine neue form medikamentoser pflaster. *Wien Med Wschr* 1896; 46:1854.

Warren R, Thayer TR. Transplantation of the saphenous vein for postphlebitic stasis. *Surgery* 1954; 35:867.

# CHAPTER 14

# Extra-anatomic bypass

*The shortest route is not the most direct one, but rather the one where the most favorable winds swell our sails.*

*(Friedrich Nietzsche)*

It was not long after Jacques Oudot's original aorta-iliac bypass that reconstruction of these vessels was recognized as an effective method of treating lower extremity ischemia. The necessity of a laparotomy and retroperitoneal dissection, however, made direct reconstruction of diseased aorta–iliac segments too hazardous for some patients. The possibility of an indirect, less invasive procedure was first conceived by Norman Freeman in 1952. In a paper describing recent advances in operations on large arteries, Freeman reported a case of left iliofemoral endarterectomy in which a right iliac artery aneurysm was noted. Cellophane was wrapped about the aneurysm, resulting in its subsequent thrombosis, and in gangrene of the right fifth toe 6 weeks later. At reoperation, Freeman divided the chronically occluded left superficial femoral artery at the adductor tendon, performed an endarterectomy, and then tunneled it into the right groin via a subcutaneous route, where an end-to-end anastomosis was performed to the divided right superficial femoral artery (Figure 14.1). The patient recovered well, with the circulation to the right foot intact. Freeman concluded:

> It is fully recognized that operative intervention does not solve the main problem –
> arteriosclerosis – since this condition is generally widespread and operation is limited
> to the particular vessel involved. However, it does give promise of relief of some of the
> complications when the disease is limited to a single vessel.

In 1958, McCaughan and Kahn reported two cases of iliac-to-contralateral popliteal crossover grafts for limb-threatening ischemia, with good results. In the first case, an anastomosis was also performed from the Dacron prosthesis to the profunda femoris of the ischemic extremity, one of the earliest uses of the sequential bypass technique. McCaughan and Kahn concluded that the procedure was safer than the usual graft from the aorta to the popliteal artery.

In 1960, Vetto attempted to render the procedure of McCaughan and Kahn safer when he used the common femoral artery, rather than the external iliac, as a donor vessel for a bypass to the contralateral extremity. In 1962, he reported a series of 10 femoral–femoral bypasses with follow-up to 16 months. Nine of the cases were successful. By 1966, Vetto had accumulated 39 cases, with continued good results, leading him to consider use of this procedure in good-risk patients as well.

Cecil Lewis of Australia developed the concept of using an upper extremity artery to supply circulation to the lower extremities. In 1959, he used a nylon

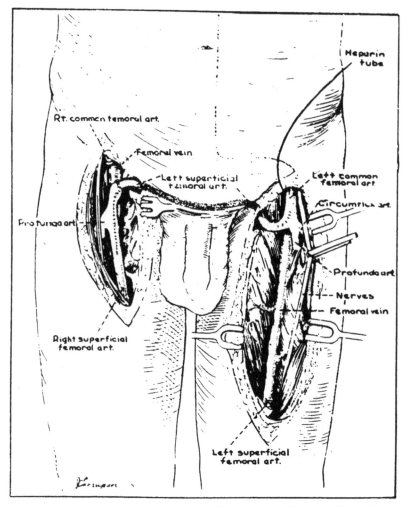

**Figure 14.1** The first femoral–femoral crossover graft (from Freeman NE, Leeds FH. Operations on large arteries. Application of recent advances. *Cal Med* 1952; 77:229).

prosthesis to construct a bypass from the subclavian artery to an aorta–iliac homograft in a case of ruptured abdominal aortic aneurysm. The patient survived and eventually returned to his occupation of greenkeeper (Figure 14.2).

The first axillary–femoral artery bypass was performed by Blaisdell in 1962, following an abdominal aortic aneurysmectomy in an elderly man who had undergone left above-knee amputation 8 years previously. On the third postoperative day, the aortic graft thrombosed, placing the right lower extremity in jeopardy. The patient was returned to the operating room and suffered cardiac arrest upon induction of anesthesia. Resuscitation was successful but because of the patient's fragile state an abdominal procedure was considered too dangerous. Blaisdell constructed a bypass from the right axillary artery to the common

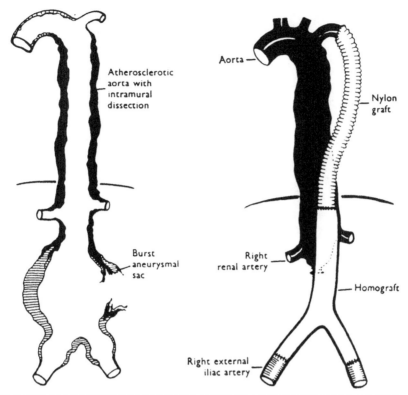

**Figure 14.2** Lower extremity blood supply derived from the subclavian artery (from Lewis CD. A subclavian artery as the means of blood-supply to the lower half of the body. *Br J Surg* 1961; 48:574).

femoral artery under local anesthesia, resulting in salvage of the patient's extremity. The Dacron prosthesis was still patent 8 months later (Figure 14.3).

Less than 1 month after Blaisdell's operation, J.H. Louw performed the identical procedure in a 52-year-old South African man with gangrenous toes.

In 1963, Blaisdell reported his use of axillary–femoral bypass in seven patients with good immediate results. Three years later, Sauvage introduced the addition of a crossover graft to the axillary–femoral for bilateral lower extremity ischemia.

Extra-anatomic bypasses were also recognized as effective alternatives to intrathoracic or mediastinal procedures, in the treatment of occlusive disease of the aortic arch and its branches. The first extrathoracic bypass was performed by Lyons and Galbraith in 1956. They used a nylon prosthesis to construct a subclavian–carotid bypass in a 67-year-old man who had internal carotid artery stenosis and transient ischemic attacks. The patient was asymptomatic 7 months after surgery. Variations of this procedure include subclavian–subclavian bypass, first performed by Ehrenfeld in 1965; and axillary–axillary bypass, introduced by Myers in 1971. Additional experiences with these procedures soon followed.

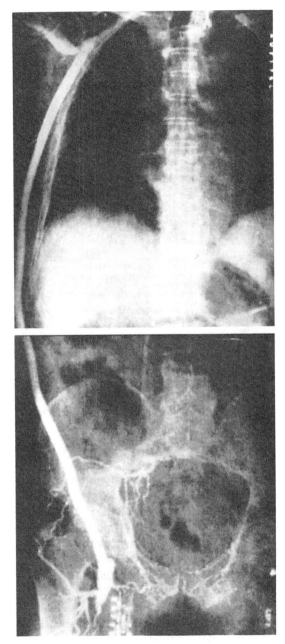

**Figure 14.3** The first axillary–femoral graft (from Blaisdell FW, Hall AD. Axillary–femoral artery bypass for lower extremity ischaemia. *Surgery* 1963; 54:563).

Dietrich reported 125 cases of subclavian–carotid bypass in 1967. In 1972 Finklestein reported 15 cases of subclavian–subclavian bypass for the subclavian steal syndrome and, by 1979, Myers had performed 18 axillary–axillary bypasses. For cases in which a cervical arterial source was unavailable, Sproul suggested femoral–axillary bypass in 1971.

The original indications for extra-anatomic bypasses were complications of aortic reconstructions, and impending limb loss in ill patients. In 1970, Parsonnet suggested that the indications for these procedures should be broadened, since they often worked well. He reported good results with 38 femoral–femoral, 11 axillary–femoral, and 10 carotid–subclavian grafts; and assuaged fears of a steal syndrome. Two years later, Parsonnet's group reported an 85 percent 5-year patency rate in 66 femoral–femoral grafts. In 1980, they reported 73 percent 5-year and 64 percent 10-year patency rates in 133 femoral–femoral grafts.

In 1977, Logerfo reported the results of 66 axillary–bifemoral and 64 axillary–femoral grafts in 120 patients. The 5-year patency rate for the former was 74 percent (20 thrombectomies in 15 grafts), versus 37 percent (25 thrombectomies in 22 grafts) for unilateral grafts. The authors concluded that axillary–bifemoral grafts had similar 5-year patency rates to aorta–iliac grafts, and were preferable to unilateral grafts owing to their superior patency rate.

In the same issue of the *Annals of Surgery* bearing Logerfo's study, more sobering results with these bypasses were reported by Eugene. One-half of his 59 axillary–femoral bypasses thrombosed within 2 years, and 47 percent of his 33 femoral–femoral bypasses closed within 4 years. He counseled that subcutaneous grafts should be performed only when an intra-abdominal procedure was contraindicated or the life expectancy was limited.

The use of "extended" extra-anatomic bypasses was reported by Veith in 1978. Twelve out of 14 axillary–popliteal bypasses were patent after 14 months. Six years later Connolly reported his results with 13 axillary–popliteal, and three axillary–tibial bypasses. Two of the former were patent after 3 years, and one of the latter was open after 18 months. In 1989, Ascer summarized the Montefiore experience, with 55 axillary–popliteal grafts performed over 12 years; the 5-year patency rate was 40 percent.

Several reports in the early 1990s renewed the debate about broadening the indications for axillary–femoral bypass. Harris found a primary patency rate of 85 percent for 76 axillary–bifemoral grafts followed for nearly 2.5 years, and concluded that more patients could be helped by this procedure.

In 1992 Schneider compared the results of 34 axillary–bifemoral and unifemoral grafts, with those of 107 aorta–femoral grafts performed synchronously. He concluded that extra-anatomic bypasses were acceptable, but hemodynamically inferior alternatives to direct reconstruction, and should be reserved for properly selected high-risk patients. One year later, El-Massry reported a primary patency rate of 73 percent for 79 axillary–femoral bypasses after 7 years, and recommended their use for incapacitating claudication as well as limb salvage.

By the millennium, most reports favored a limited role for extra-anatomic bypasses, reserving them for critically ill patients unable to tolerate direct aortic reconstructions. Advances in anesthesiology, cardiology, and critical care medicine have significantly reduced the number of these patients.

## Bibliography

Alpert J, Brief DK, Parsonnet V. Vascular restoration for aortoiliac occlusion and an alternative approach to the poor risk patient. *J Newark Beth Israel Hosp* 1967; 18:4.

Ascer E, Veith FJ, Gupta S. Axillofemoral bypass grafting: indications, late results, and determinants of long-term patency. *J Vasc Surg* 1989; 10:285.

Blaisdell FW, Hall AD. Axillary-femoral artery bypass for lower extremity ischemia. *Surgery* 1963; 54:563.

Brief DK, Alpert J, Parsonnet V. Crossover femorofemoral grafts: compromise or preference: A reappraisal. *Arch Surg* 1972; 105:889.

Brief DK, Brener BJ, Alpert J, et al. Crossover femorofemoral grafts followed up five years or more. *Arch Surg* 1975; 110:1294.

Connolly JE, Kwaan JHM, Brownell D, et al. Newer developments of extraanatomic bypass. *Surg Gynecol Obstet* 1984; 158:415.

Criado E, Burnham SJ, Tinsley EA Jr., et al. Femorofemoral bypass graft: analysis of patency and factors influencing long term outcome. *J Vasc Surg* 1993; 18:495.

Dick LS, Brief DK, Alpert J, et al. A 12 year experience with femorofemoral crossover grafts. *Arch Surg* 1980; 115:1359.

Diethrich EB, Garrett HE, Ameriso J, et al. Occlusive disease of the common carotid and subclavian arteries treated by carotid-subclavian bypass. Analysis of 125 cases. *Am J Surg* 1967; 114:800.

Donaldson MC, Louras JC, Bucknam CA. Axillofemoral bypass: A tool with a limited role. *J Vasc Surg* 1986; 3:757.

Ehrenfeld WK, Levin SM, Wylie EJ. Venous crossover bypass grafts for arterial insufficiency. *Ann Surg* 1968; 167:287.

El-Massry S, Saad E, Sauvage LR, et al. Axillofemoral bypass using externally-supported, knitted Dacron grafts: a follow-up through twelve years. *J Vasc Surg* 1993; 17:107.

Eugene J, Goldstone J, Moore WS. Fifteen-year experience with subcutaneous bypass grafts for lower extremity ischemia. *Ann Surg* 1976; 186:177.

Finkelstein NM, Byer A, Rush BF Jr. Subclavian-subclavian bypass for the subclavian steal syndrome. *Surgery* 1972; 71:142.

Freeman NE, Leeds FH. Operations on large arteries. Application of recent advances. *Cal Med* 1952; 77:229.

Harris EJ, Taylor LM, McConnell DB, et al. Clinical results of axillobifemoral bypass using externally supported polytetrafluoroethylene. *J Vasc Surg* 1990; 12:416.

Illuminati G, Calio PG, Mangialardi N, et al. Results of axillofemoral by-passes for aorto-iliac occlusive disease. *Langenbecks Arch Surg* 1996; 381:212.

Johnson WC, LoGerfo FW, Vollman RW. Is axillobilateral femoral graft an effective substitute for aortobilateral iliac femoral graft? *Ann Surg* 1976; 186:123.

Keller MP, Hoch JR, Harding AD, et al. Axillopopliteal bypass for limb salvage. *J Vasc Surg* 1992; 15:817.

Lewis CD. A subclavian artery as the means of blood-supply to the lower half of the body. *Br J Surg* 1961; 48:574.

LoGerfo FW, Johnson WC, Corson JD, *et al*. A comparison of the late patency rates of axillobilat-eral femoral and axillounilateral femoral grafts. *Surgery* 1977; 81:33.

Louw JH. Splenic-to-femoral and axillary-to-femoral bypass grafts in diffuse atherosclerotic occlusive disease. *Lancet* 1963; 1:1401.

Lyons C, Galbraith G. Surgical treatment of atherosclerotic occlusion of the internal carotid artery. *Ann Surg* 1957; 146:487.

McCaughan JJ Jr., Kahn SF. Cross-over graft for unilateral occlusive disease of the iliofemoral arteries. *Ann Surg* 1960; 151:26.

Mannick JA, Williams LE, Nabseth DC. The late results of axillofemoral grafts. *Surgery* 1970; 68:1038.

Myers WO, Lawton BR, Sautter RD. Axillo-axillary bypass graft. *JAMA* 1971; 217:826.

Myers WO, Lawton BR, Ray JF III, *et al*. Axillo-axillary bypass for subclavian steal syndrome. *Arch Surg* 1979; 114:394.

Parsonnet V, Alpert J, Brief DK. Femorofemoral and axillofemoral grafts: compromise or preference? *Surgery* 1970; 67:26.

Passman MA, Taylor LM, Moneta GL, *et al*. Comparison of axillofemoral and aortofemoral bypass for aortoiliac occlusive disease. *J Vasc Surg* 1996; 23:263.

Plecha FR, Plecha FM. Femorofemoral bypass grafts: Ten-year experience. *J Vasc Surg* 1984; 1:555.

Posner MP, Riles TS, Ramirez AA, *et al*. Axilloaxillary bypass for symptomatic stenosis of the subclavian artery. *Am J Surg* 1983; 145:644.

Rutherford RB, Patt A, Pearce WH. Extra-anatomic bypass: a closer view. *J Vasc Surg* 1987; 5:437.

Sauvage LR, Wood SJ. Unilateral axillary bilateral femoral bifurcation graft: A procedure for the poor risk patient with aortoiliac disease. *Surgery* 1966; 60:573.

Schanzer H, Chung-Loy H, Kotok M, *et al*. Evaluation of axillo-axillary artery bypass for the treatment of subclavian or innominate artery occlusive disease. *J Cardiovasc Surg* 1987; 28:258.

Schneider JR, McDaniel MD, Walsh DB, *et al*. Axillofemoral bypass: outcome and hemody-namic results in high-risk patients. *J Vasc Surg* 1992; 15:952.

Veith FJ, Moss CM, Daly V, *et al*. New approaches to limb salvage by extended extra-anatomic bypasses and prosthetic reconstructions to foot arteries. *Surgery* 1978; 84:764.

Vetto RM. The treatment of unilateral iliac artery obstruction with a transabdominal, subcuta-neous, femorofemoral graft. *Surgery* 1962; 52:342.

Vetto RM. The femorofemoral shunt. An appraisal. *Am J Surg* 1966; 112:162.

Vetto RM, Dunphy JE. Recent revisions in the operative treatment of vascular disease. *Surg Gynecol Obstet* 1964; 119:1026.

Ziomek S, Quinones-Baldrich WJ, Busuttil RW, *et al*. The superiority of synthetic arterial grafts over autogenous veins in carotid-subclavian bypass. *J Vasc Surg* 1986; 3:140.

PART 6

# The French connection

# CHAPTER 15

# Mathieu Jaboulay

*It is common sense to take a method and try it. If it fails, admit it frankly and try another. But above all, try something.*

*(Franklin D. Roosevelt)*

Mathieu Jaboulay was born in France in 1860 and was the first in a succession of French surgeons that limned most of the basic concepts in vascular surgery. As a surgeon in Lyon, Jaboulay was fascinated by the report of arterial suturing by Jassinowsky, in 1891, and several years later by Heidenhain. These prompted him to begin the first experiments in France, on arterial suturing. He was assisted by his intern, Eugèbe Briau.

In 1892, Jaboulay was named Head Surgeon at the Hotel-Dieu. Four years later, Briau and Jaboulay published the first French article on vascular surgery in *Lyon Médicale*. They described their results with circular anastomoses and carotid interposition grafts in dogs. All of the arteries thrombosed within 4 days. Undaunted, Jaboulay revised his technique by everting the arterial edges. With better results he concluded:

> The arterial graft will give us the means to combat gangrene of arterial origin against which we are helpless. The treatment of aneurysms and arterial contusions will be transformed.

Jaboulay also correctly predicted the use of this technique in the venous system. He speculated about placing venous autografts into the arterial system and predicted that this would replace the ligature as a treatment for arterial injuries.

In 1901, Jaboulay advised Carrel and Morel to attempt carotid–jugular anastomoses in dogs, as a means of improving cerebral circulation. Carrel obtained good results, with beating subcutaneous jugular veins after 3 weeks. These results were also reported in *Lyon Médicale*, in 1902.

In 1906, Mathieu Jaboulay carried out the first attempts at human kidney transplantation. On January 22, he transplanted a porcine kidney to the brachial vessels of a woman suffering from nephrotic syndrome. Three months later, he repeated this treatment in a different patient, with a goat kidney. Neither of the xenografts lasted more than several hours and both had to be excised. Jaboulay was unfazed by these failures and concluded:

> If these grafts become feasible, no area of the body will know better how to employ it than the bend of the elbow for ease and mildness of operating maneuvers.

The pinnacle of Jaboulay's career was reached in 1902, when he became Chairman of the Surgical Clinic at the Hotel-Dieu. Jaboulay held this post until his death in 1913. While traveling to Paris to examine applicants for ophthalmology positions at a local university, he died in a train accident in Melun.

## Bibliography

Bouchet A. Les pionniers Lyonnais de la chirurgie vasculaire: M. Jaboulay, A. Carrel, E. Villard et R Leriche. *Hist Sci Med* 1994; 28:223.

Jaboulay M. Le traitement de quelques troubles trophiques du pied et de la jambe par la denudation de l'artère fémorale et la distension des nerfs vasculaires. *Lyon Méd* 1899; 91:467.

Jaboulay M. Chirurgie des artères. *Semin Méd* 1902: 405.

Jaboulay M. Greffe du rein au pli du coude par soudure artérielle et veineuse. *Lyon Méd* 1906; 107:575.

Jaboulay M, Briau E. Recherches expérimentales sur la suture et la greffe artérielle. *Lyon Méd* 1896; 81:97.

# CHAPTER 16

# Eugène Villard

*Curiosity is, in great and generous minds, the first passion and the last.*

(Samuel Johnson)

Eugène Villard was born in France in 1868. Inspired by the work of Carrel in the United States, and by a slew of Lyonese theses dedicated to vascular surgery (Louis Bérard, 1909; Pierre Charnois, 1909; Emile Perrin, 1911) Villard began experimenting with vascular and renal grafts in 1910. He collaborated with fellow surgeons Louis Tavernier and Emile Perrin, and relied upon Delachanal and Dubreuil for histologic examination of specimens. After 4 years of experimental surgery in Lyon, their results were presented at the New York International Convention of Surgery, in 1914.

Regarding autogenous carotid arterial grafts in dogs Villard wrote: "The arteries implanted in the same animals formed scar tissue without modification."

In another series of experiments, canine iliac arteries were grafted onto the carotid arteries of other dogs. The grafts were harvested 12 days later and examined microscopically by Dubreuil, who concluded: "The histologic structure is so perfectly preserved that it is impossible to distinguish where the graft was cut."

Villard and his colleagues also performed numerous autogenous venous grafts in dogs with continuous failures in the early period. Eventually, however, they succeeded in replacing a carotid artery with external jugular vein. The graft was examined after nearly 4 months and found to be in perfect condition. Villard offered an early description of neointimal fibrous hyperplasia:

> The vascular wall thickening, which shows up especially in the middle membrane, is made up for the most part of neoformations of a smooth muscular type. To synthesize in a word these histologic modifications, one could say that the venous graft implanted on an artery truly makes itself an artery.

Villard also experimented with grafts preserved by freezing, but most of his grafts thrombosed. Among the few successes were three carotid homografts, and a human saphenous vein graft implanted into a feline abdominal aorta. Villard was pessimistic about the prospects for preserved grafts, unless the technique for preservation could be improved.

Villard distinguished himself as a great teacher and in 1921 became Chairman of Operating Medicine, in Lyon. From 1925 to 1927 he was also the Chairman of the Gynecology Clinic.

Eugène Villard died in 1953.

## Bibliography

Bouchet A. Les pionniers Lyonnais de la chirurgie vasculaire: M. Jaboulay, A. Carrel, E. Villard et R Leriche. *Hist Sci Med* 1994; 28:223.

Villard E. *Greffes vasculaires*. XIVe Congrès international de Chirurgie, New York, April 1914.

Villard E, Perrin E. Greffes vasculaires. *Lyon Chir* 1912; 8:267.

Villard E, Perrin E. Traitement des obliterations vasculaires. *Lyon Chir* 1913; 9:4.

Villard E, Tavernier L, Perrin E. Recherches expérimentales sur les greffes vasculaires. *Lyon Chir* 1911; 6:144.

# CHAPTER 17

# Alexis Carrel

*To yield to every whim of curiosity, and to allow our passion for inquiry to be restrained by nothing but the limits of our ability, this shows an eagerness of mind not unbecoming to scholarship. But it is wisdom that has the merit of selecting from among the innumerable problems which present themselves, those whose solution is important to mankind.*

*(Immanuel Kant)*

Historians of every field seek an individual upon whom to fix the epithet "Father." In vascular surgery, the search ends upon review of the life and contributions of Alexis Carrel, whose extraordinary imagination and foresight suggest a parallel to the vision of his more celebrated countryman, Jules Verne (Figure 17.1). Many decades prior to their invention, Verne accurately predicted the use of airplanes, submarines, television, guided missiles, and space satellites. His well-known tales have carried readers under, above, and around the earth. Carrel foresaw the routine suturing of blood vessels and use of vein bypass grafts; reimplantation of severed limbs; the preservation and transplantation of kidneys, thyroid, heart, and lung; and cardiac valvular reconstruction and extracorporeal circulation. Unlike Verne's imaginings, however, Carrel's were realized in his own lifetime.

Carrel was born in Lyon, France, in 1873. When Carrel was 5 years old, his father died, and the responsibility of helping to care for a younger brother and sister had an early maturing effect. Alexis was a very quiet, serious child and attended St. Joseph's Day School, an institution administered by Jesuit priests.

Carrel showed little interest in music and art and spent most of his free time reading. In 1889, he received a Baccalaureate in Letters, and one in Science the following year. After graduation, Carrel enrolled in the medical school at the University of Lyon. Following 3 years there, he became an extern at the Red Cross Hospital and the Hôpital Antiguaille.

In 1895, Carrel fulfilled 1 year of military service with the French mountain troops and spent the next 5 years completing his internship in several hospitals throughout Lyon.

At this time there was little work being done in the field of vascular surgery. In 1896, Mathieu Jaboulay, a teacher of Carrel during his internship, published one of the first papers describing end-to-end anastomosis of blood vessels. In the United States, John Murphy would soon describe his repair of a lacerated femoral artery and in Germany Edwin Payr was conducting preliminary experiments substituting magnesium tubes for arterial segments. Vascular surgery was, therefore, barely in its infancy when an event occurred that altered the life of Carrel and hastened the age of routine operation on the heart and blood vessels.

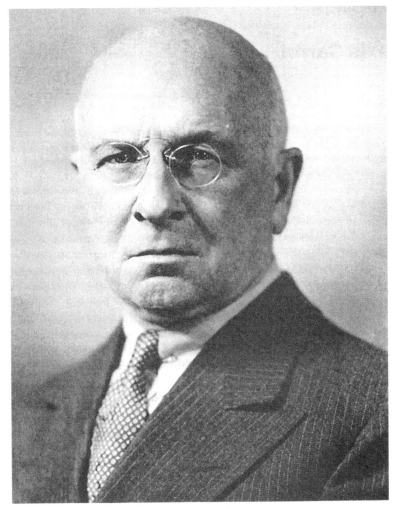

**Figure 17.1** Alexis Carrel (courtesy of the Rockefeller University Archives).

In 1894, the President of the French Republic was Sadi Carnot. While in Lyon, he suffered a stab wound to the abdomen at the hands of an Italian anarchist. The blade severed the portal vein and, in accordance with the prevailing notions of the day, the best surgeons in France threw up their hands in frustration, convinced that nothing could be done to save their President.

Carrel was deeply moved by the death of Carnot and could not accept the helplessness of Carnot's surgeons. Carrel was emphatic in his belief that if surgeons were able to repair blood vessels as they could skin and other tissues, Carnot would have been saved.

In 1899, mindful of Jaboulay's attempts at uniting blood vessels, Carrel began his first experiments in the laboratory of Mariel Soulier, a professor of therapeutics. Most of these involved construction of arterial–venous fistulas in canine necks, between the external jugular vein and carotid artery. Carrel developed new sutures and needles for this work and he also received embroidery lessons to which he later ascribed his manual dexterity.

At the turn of the century, it was necessary to pass a difficult clinical examination to gain a surgical faculty position in Lyon. Most students required several attempts to pass and by 1903, Carrel had failed twice. That same year Carrel accompanied a pilgrimage to Lourdes, where miraculous cures were said to occur. There he encountered a young girl dying of tuberculous peritonitis. Unconscious and deemed too ill to undergo the usual immersion in the curative pool, she was sprinkled with a few of its drops. The girl regained consciousness within a few hours and went on to make a miraculous recovery. She became a nun and lived for 34 more years. Carrel was mystified by these events and chose to credit the power of suggestion as the only rational explanation. He nonetheless faithfully reported what he had witnessed, and was attacked by clergy and medical colleagues alike upon his return to Lyon: by the one contingent for his skepticism and by the other for his gullibility. Informed that he now had no chance of passing his surgical examination, he contemplated leaving France and medicine altogether.

In May 1904, Carrel left France for Montreal. Several months later he presented a paper on vascular anastomosis to the Second Medical Congress of the French Language of North America. It was well received by the audience, of which Karl Beck, a respected Chicago surgeon, was a member. Beck approached Carrel with the possibility of working in the United States and, in August 1904, Carrel began a 2-month trek west across Canada, south through California, then east to Chicago. He eventually accepted a position at the University of Chicago in the Physiology Department under the chairmanship of Dr George Stuart.

Carrel was assigned to work with Charles Claude Guthrie, a young physiologist who had graduated from medical school 4 years earlier. Between November 1904 and August 1906, the two shared one of the most productive relationships in the history of medicine. During these 21 months, 9 of which Guthrie spent at the University of Missouri on sabbatical, they wrote 28 papers together. Carrel added five more of his own and Guthrie two. Their experimental work included perfection of vascular anastomoses and the use of vein grafts in the arterial system; development of tissue preservation techniques; reimplantation of limbs and transplantation of kidneys, ovaries, thyroids, and hearts.

Carrel's vision would be realized in the first routine use of saphenous vein bypasses in 1948, the first successful human renal transplant in 1955, and the performance of the first human limb reimplantation in 1962. Christian Barnard would perform the first human heart transplant in 1967, 62 years after Carrel's description.

The collaboration of these two great men ended in 1906, when Guthrie accepted a position as Professor of Physiology and Pharmacology at Washington University in St. Louis. Carrel was disappointed by the lack of financial support for his research so he moved to the Rockefeller Institute in New York (Figure 17.2).

Carrel began his work in the Experimental Surgical Department of the Rockefeller Institute by continuing his investigations of preserved vascular homografts to replace segments of cat abdominal aortas. During the next 4 years, he improved preservation techniques for transplantation of carotid arteries from one dog to another. Carrel performed experiments on the thoracic aorta, interposing vena cava grafts and using paraffin tubes as shunts to prevent spinal cord ischemia.

In a paper presented to the American Surgical Association in 1910, Carrel described mitral valvulotomy and annuloplasty, ventricular aneurysmectomy, and coronary artery bypass. His fame was also growing as a result of his contributions to the field of tissue culture (Figure 17.3). Carrel's meticulous application of aseptic techniques and his fine dexterity were responsible for his successes in this field, just as they had been in vascular surgery.

For his hitherto unparalleled accomplishments in vascular surgery and organ transplantation, Alexis Carrel was awarded the Nobel Prize for Physiology and Medicine in October 1912. It is alleged that Carrel learned of the award while browsing through a New York morning paper. Carrel was the youngest scientist, as well as the first United States scientist, to earn this prize. At a ceremony in his honor, President William Taft pronounced:

> The names of Harvey Pasteur, Walter Reed, Koch, are great names which share the progress toward a superior knowledge of the human and of medicine, and from now on, Dr. Carrel will take his place among them.

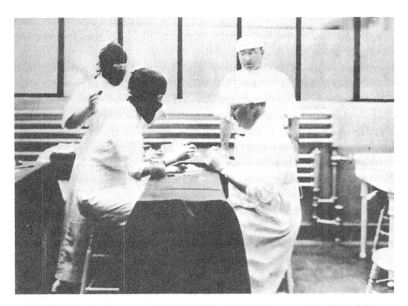

**Figure 17.2** Carrel's operating room at the Rockefeller Institute (courtesy of the Rockefeller University Archives).

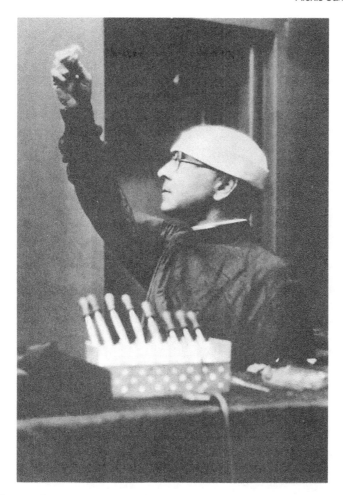

**Figure 17.3** Examination of tissue cultures by Carrel (courtesy of the Rockefeller University Archives).

In 1913, Alexis Carrel was made Knight of the Legion of Honor by the French government. In the latter part of that year he married a long-time friend, Ann Marie de la Meyrei.

When World War I broke out, Carrel was vacationing in France. As a French citizen he was bound to serve his country when ordered to report to Lyon (Figure 17.4). The terrible infections spawned on the battlefields of Europe during this conflict rekindled Carrel's interest in wound healing.

Carrel sought ways to treat advanced infections and through contacts at the Rockefeller Institute he was introduced to a chemist named Henry Dakin. After testing hundreds of antiseptic solutions, the two devised a means of irrigating wounds with the solution that still bears Dakin's name and remains in common use.

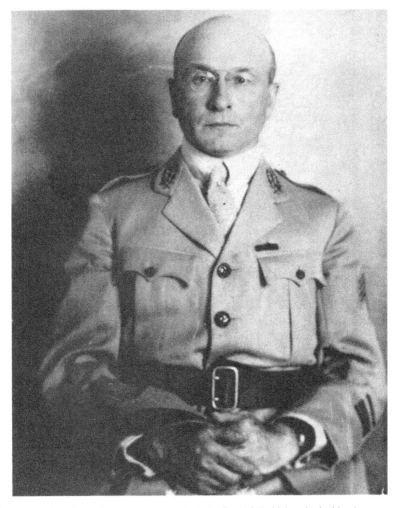

**Figure 17.4** Carrel in the French Army (courtesy of the Rockefeller University Archives).

In 1915, Carrel became Commander in the French Army's Legion of Honor. In the following year, he received the Order of Leopold from King Albert of Belgium. Carrel also received the Order of the Northern Star of Sweden and was made a companion of the Order of St. Michael and St. George.

In 1917, the first mobile army hospital was opened under Carrel's direction. This was a forerunner of the MASH units that would play a vital role in Korea and Vietnam, and contribute significantly to the advancement of vascular surgery.

Following the war, Carrel returned to New York and devoted his attention to development of a perfusion pump for organ preservation. He was introduced to the great aviator Charles Lindbergh, who professed a similar interest following the severe respiratory illness of a relative affecting the heart. Working together, they constructed a Pyrex pump in 1935 that sustained a cat thyroid gland for 18 days. Preservation of hearts, ovaries, fallopian tubes, spleens, kidneys, and pancreases soon followed. The Lindbergh pump provided the groundwork for eventual development of modern pump oxygenators and the mechanical heart (Figure 17.5).

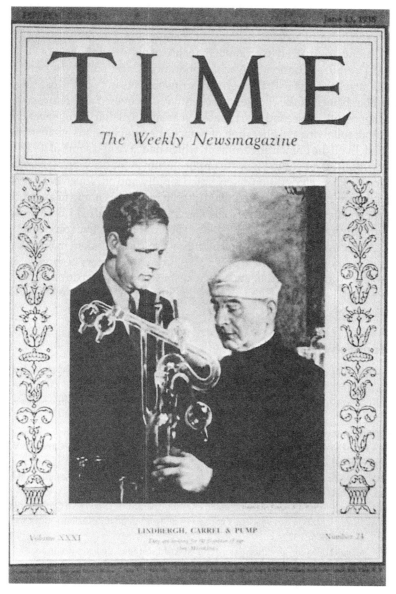

**Figure 17.5** Charles Lindbergh and Alexis Carrel with their perfusion pump, on the cover of *TIME* magazine, June 13, 1938 (reprinted by permission from *TIME*).

In 1939, Carrel was forced into mandatory retirement from the Rockefeller Institute; he was 65. His bitterness gave rise to denunciation of the Institute and of science in general. Carrel and his wife left the United States and returned to France.

During the early 1940s, Carrel devoted himself to the creation of an "Institute of Man," the realization of a long-held dream. In 1941, the "Fondation Francaise Pour l'Etude des Problemes Humains" was sanctioned by law and charged with: ". . . researching all practical solutions and proceeding with all demonstrations in view of improving the physiological, mental, and social condition of the population." Carrel eschewed all political issues and functions during World War II, preferring instead to promote the cause of his foundation.

In 1943, amid accusations of Nazi collaboration, Carrel suffered his first heart attack. Carrel had met with the Germans to insure the safety of his Institute, and this probably incited the charges. He eventually recovered and returned to the foundation until his second heart attack 1 year later. This left Carrel severely disabled and, following the liberation of France, the vituperations against him intensified. Even the French government, which had lavished some of its greatest honors upon Carrel, sought ways to implicate him in the German nightmare.

Carrel's physical condition deteriorated rapidly, and on November 5, 1944, at 8 p.m., French radio broadcasted that Carrel had fled his home to avoid being tried for collaborating with the Nazis. Carrel had, in fact, died 9 hours prior to this radio message. Proof of the alleged collaboration was never produced.

The tragic events of Carrel's final months were a bitter denouement to the life of one of the most ingenious and prescient figures in the history of surgery. There are few innovations in cardiac and vascular surgery today that do not have roots in his work. The epithet "Father of Vascular Surgery" is justly applied to Alexis Carrel.

## Bibliography

Baader W, Nyhus LM. The life of Carl Beck and an important interval with Alexis Carrel. *Surg Gynecol Obstet* 1986; 163:85.

Barnard CN. What we have learned about heart transplantations. *J Thorac Cardiovasc Surg* 1968; 56:457.

Bing RJ. Carrel. A personal reminiscence. *JAMA* 1983; 250:3297.

Bouchet A. Les pionniers Lyonnais de la chirurgie vasculaire: M. Jaboulay, A. Carrel, E. Villard et R Leriche. *Hist Sci Med* 1994; 28:223.

Carrel A. La technique opératiore des anastomoses vasculaires et la transplantation des viscères. *Lyon Méd* 1902; 98:88.

Carrel A. Les anastomoses vasculares et leur technique opératoire. *Union Med Can* 1904; 33:521.

Carrel A. Transplantation des vaisseaux conserves au froid pendant plusieurs jours. *Comptes Rendu Soc Biol* 1906; 2:57.

Carrel A. Au sujet de la conservation des artères en "cold storage." *Comptes Rendu Soc Biol* 1907; 62:1178.

Carrel A. Résultats éloignés de la transplantation des veines sur les artères. *Rev Chir* 1910; XVL:987.

Carrel A. On the experimental surgery of the thoracic aorta and the heart. *Ann Surg* 1910; 52:83.

Carrel A. Graft of the vena cava on the abdominal aorta. *Ann Surg* 1910; 52:462.

Carrel A. The preservation of tissues and its applications in surgery. *JAMA* 1912; 59:523.

Carrel A. Experimental operations on the orifices of the heart. *Ann Surg* 1914; 60:1.

Carrel A. Experimental operations on the sigmoid valves of the pulmonary artery. *J Exp Med* 1914; 20:9.

Carrel A. Present condition of a strain of connective tissue twenty-eight months old. *J Exp Med* 1914; 20:1.

Carrel A, Burrows MT. Human sarcoma cultivated outside of the body. *JAMA* 1910; 55:1732.

Carrel A, Guthrie CC. The transplantation of veins and organs. *Am Med* 1905; 10:1101.

Carrel A, Guthrie CC. Uniterminal and biterminal venous transplantations. *Surg Gynecol Obstet* 1906; 2:266.

Carrel A, Lindbergh CA. *The Culture of Organs*. New York: Paul B. Hoeber, Inc., 1938.

Carrel A, Morel. Anastomose bout à bout de la jugulaire et de la carotide primitive. *Lyon Méd* 1902; 99:1.

Carrel A, Morel. Présentation d'un chien porteur d'une anastomose artério-veineuse. *Lyon Méd* 1902; 99:152.

Carrel A, Moullard J. Anastomose bout à bout de la jugulaire et de la carotide primitive. *Lyon Med* 1902; 99:114.

Carrel A, Dakin H, Daufresne J, *et al*. Traitement abortif de l'infection des plaies. *Bull Acad Med Paris* 1915; 76:361.

Edwards WS, Edwards PD. *Alexis Carrel, Visionary Surgeon*. Springfield: Charles C. Thomas, 1974.

Hallowell C. Charles Lindbergh. *Am Heritage Inv Tech* 1985; Fall:58.

Hardy JD. Transplantation of blood vessels, organs and limbs. *JAMA* 1983; 250:954.

Jaboulay M, Briau E. Recherches expérimentales sur la suture et la greffe artérielles. *Lyon Med* 1896; 81:97.

Kunlin J. Le traitement de l'artèrite oblitérante par la greffe veineuse. *Arch Mal Coeur* 1949; 42:371.

Malt RA, McKhann CF. Replantation of severed arms. *JAMA* 1964; 189:716.

Murphy JB. Resection of arteries and veins injured in continuity – End-to-end suture – Experimental and clinical research. *Med Rec* 1897; 51:73.

Murray JE, Merrill JP, Harrison JH. Renal homotransplantation in identical twins. *Surg Forum* 1955; 6:432.

Najafi H. Dr. Alexis Carrel and tissue culture. *JAMA* 1983; 250:1086.

Payr E. Zur frage der circulaeren vereingung von blutgefaessen mit resorbibaren prothesen. *Arch Klin Chir* 1900; 62:67.

Shaw R, Stubenbord WT. Alexis Carrel MD. Contribution to kidney transplantation and preservation. *NY State J Med* 1980; 8:1438.

Tuffier T, Carrel A. Patching and section of the pulmonary orifice of the heart. *J Exp Med* 1914; 20:3.

# CHAPTER 18

# René Leriche

*A teacher can but lead you to the door; learning is up to you.*

*(Chinese proverb)*

René Leriche was born in October 1879 in Roanne, France. As a boy, he dreamed of becoming a soldier, but eventually he developed an interest in medicine. He attended medical school at the University of Lyon and received his degree in 1906. His thesis was entitled "The Surgical Treatment of Cancer of the Stomach." Leriche's choice of surgery was influenced by his contact with several of the field's luminaries. Mathieu Jaboulay was one of his instructors, Leriche had several opportunities to assist Antonin Poncet with surgery, and Alexis Carrel was a chief resident when Leriche was a medical student. Leriche and Carrel worked together for 6 months and they resided in the same boarding house. Leriche was always grateful to Carrel for his friendship and for teaching him the importance of observation.

Carrel left France in 1904 and continually encouraged Leriche to visit other countries. Leriche eventually arrived in the United States while Carrel was at the Rockefeller Institute. In New York Leriche met Simon Flexner and visited the Roosevelt and German hospitals; in Chicago he met John Murphy and Evarts Graham; and in Boston he met Harvey Cushing. The highlight of his trip, however, was several days spent with William Halstead in Baltimore.

Carrel continued to pressure Leriche into emigrating to the United States. In 1914, Leriche was on the verge of doing so when World War I began. Leriche remained in France and became a surgeon at La Houleuse camp, where wounded soldiers were cared for. Leriche gained much experience in treating skeletal, and central and peripheral nerve injuries, and here his interest in the sympathetic nervous system and various pain syndromes began. He received accolades from the French and Belgian governments for his work during the war.

In 1917, Leriche and Jean Heitz demonstrated the benefits of arteriectomy before the Society of Biology. They proposed that resection of an obstructed artery resulted in "reheating" of the extremity and the disappearance of pain, cyanosis, and edema. Leriche also described ulcer healing from arteriectomy.

In 1924, at the age of 45, Leriche became Professor of Clinical Surgery at Strasbourg, succeeding Louis Sencert. He directed a large surgical service at the Hôpital Civil, one of the oldest in Europe. Leriche distinguished himself by his physiologic approach to surgery, also espoused by Cushing and Halstead in the United States. He was particularly interested in the vasomotor, humoral, and hematologic consequences of surgery.

Leriche's Alsatian period lasted 8 years. In 1932, he returned to Lyon to become Chairman of External Pathology and surgeon at the Hotel-Dieu. During

the inauguration of the new Grange-Blanche hospital the following year,
Edouard Herriot, the mayor of Lyon, honored Leriche as a pioneer in surgery.
Ever restless, Leriche soon returned to Strasbourg for 2 more years. In 1936, he
replaced Charles Nicolle as Professor of Experimental Medicine at the Collège
de France. Leriche's annual Chairman's lectures were eventually published in
*The Surgery of Pain*. The book enjoyed several editions and multiple translations.
Leriche had no clinical service in Paris, and operated instead at the American
Hospital in Neuilly.

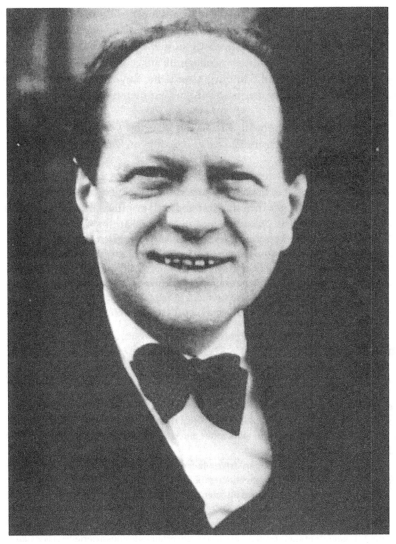

**Figure 18.1**  René Leriche (from Callow AD. Historical development of vascular grafts. In: Sawyer
PN, Kaplitt MJ, eds. *Vascular Grafts*. New York: Appleton-Century-Crofts, 1978).

During World War II, Leriche returned to Lyon, where he directed Pavilion G of the Edouard Herriot Hospital. He described the syndrome that bears his name in *Presse Médicale*, in 1940, although his earlier ruminations on this subject appeared in 1923. Leriche speculated that: "the ideal treatment would be to remove the occluded zone and reestablish arterial patency." He also added his doubt, however, that this would ever be possible.

After the liberation of France, Leriche returned to the Collège de France where he began a laboratory of experimental surgery with Jean Kunlin. Leriche was elected a member of the Academy of Sciences in 1945 and he retired from practice 5 years later (Figure 18.1).

In 1951, he became president of the International Society of Surgery and published another book, *The Philosophy of Surgery*. Leriche eventually published well over 1000 papers on all aspects of surgery and physiology. He was an honorary fellow of the American College of Surgeons, the Royal College of Surgeons of England and Edinburgh, and the Royal Society of Medicine. Leriche received honorary doctorates from 13 universities, including Glasgow and Harvard.

Leriche became severely ill during the last few years of his life and he returned to Cassis, in the south of France. He died on December 28, 1955, at the age of 76.

It is ironic that, despite Leriche's many contributions to the physiology and philosophy of surgery, he resolutely turned his back on reconstructive arterial surgery. Kunlin dared perform the first femoral–popliteal bypass in 1948 only when Leriche was absent. Nevertheless, of Leriche, Kunlin wrote:

> He was for 30 years the head of an exceptional school for surgery, for he combined a very fertile imagination with a vast clinical experience from which he drew simple and clear rules. The generations of physicians that he trained still remember him, for his lessons were accompanied by striking examples. Patient rounds were a feast for the mind, for they were often the occasion for a springing of extraordinary new ideas. Certain were adopted, others were taken up again later, for at the time they were too advanced.

## Bibliography

Bouchet A. Les pionniers Lyonnais de la chirurgie vasculaire: M. Jaboulay, A. Carrel, E. Villard et R Leriche. *Hist Sci Med* 1994; 28:223.

Jarrett F. René Leriche (1879–1955): Father of vascular surgery. *Surgery* 1979; 86:736.

Kieny R. René Leriche and his work as time goes by. *Ann Vasc Surg* 1990; 4:105.

Kunlin J. Traitement de l'artérite oblitérante par la greffe veineuse. *Arch Mal Coeur* 1949, 371.

Leriche R. De la sympathectomie péri-artérielle et de ses resultants. *Presse Méd* 1917; 25:513.

Leriche R. Des obliterations artérielles hautes (oblitération de la terminaison de l'aorte) comme cause des insuffisances circlatoires des membres inférueurs. *Bull Mém Soc Chir (Paris)* 1923; 49:1404.

Leriche R. Considération sur certaines types d'artérites oblitérantes, sur la claudication intermittente bilatérale et sur le traitement précoce de certaines lesions artérielles. *Lyon Chir* 1925; 22:521.

Leriche R. Données générales sur l'artérite oblitérante juvenile. Résultat de leur traitement par l'artériectomie et la surrénalectomie. *Bull Mém Soc Chir (Paris)* 1928; 54:201.

Leriche R. De la resection du carrefour aorto-illiaque avec double sympathectomie lombaire pour thrombose aortique. Le syndrome de l'oblitération termino-aortique par artérite. *Press Méd* 1940; 486:1.

Leriche R, Morel A. Considèrations sur le traitement des arterites et des embolies artérielles. *Lyon Méd* 1933; 151:393.

Leriche R, Stricker P. *Artéruectinue dans les Artérites Oblitérantes.* Paris: Masson, 1933:198.

Wertheimer P. L'œuvre de René Leriche. *Lyon Chir* 1956; 52:21.

# CHAPTER 19

# Jean Kunlin

*No one ever approaches perfection except by stealth, and unknown to themselves.*
*(William Hazlitt)*

Jean Kunlin was born in Schitigheim, near Strasbourg, on July 7, 1904. He studied medicine in Strasbourg, where he was an intern, and then an assistant to René Leriche. Kunlin's career began in Leriche's laboratory of experimental surgery, in Mount Saint Martin's Hospital. There he met Cid Dos Santos, Malan, DeBakey, and many other pioneers in vascular surgery. It was the concept of thromboendarterectomy, originated by Joao Cid Dos Santos (son of Reynaldo) that sparked the imagination of Kunlin. Kunlin and Cid Dos Santos had spent time together in Leriche's laboratory in 1935.

Prior to World War II, Kunlin was Chief Surgeon of the Hôpital Meurthe et Moselle. When the war began, Kunlin moved to Paris and met up again with Leriche. Kunlin pursued a dual role as practicing surgeon at the American Hospital, and as a researcher at the College de France, and then the Val de Grace. In the laboratory, his interests included extracorporeal circulation, gas embolism, venous reconstructive surgery, microanastomoses (1–2 mm vessels), and other aspects of vascular surgery. Some of these techniques were eventually used for portal–caval shunts and distal lower extremity vein grafts in humans.

In 1947, Cid Dos Santos traveled to Paris to be reunited with Leriche and Kunlin. He demonstrated his revolutionary thromboendarterectomy, and attributed his success to the use of heparin. Surgeons in Paris began performing this procedure, and Kunlin sought ways to improve it in the laboratory. His initial attempts at modifying the suturing technique were unsuccessful, and he attributed this to the absence of the endothelium. These failures undoubtedly prompted Kunlin to attempt the first saphenous vein bypass.

In 1948, Kunlin was still collaborating with Leriche in the experimental surgery laboratory of the Collège de France, and at the American hospital where the department of surgery had 11 beds. It was here that Kunlin encountered a 54-year-old man with a 3-month history of ischemic rest pain. The patient had undergone a great-toe amputation, which led to gangrene of the dorsal surface of the foot. A lumbar sympathectomy and femoral arteriectomy had already been performed, precluding endarterectomy. An arteriogram revealed a patent popliteal artery with posterior tibial runoff. Kunlin proposed a femoral–popliteal bypass with saphenous vein; Leriche proposed continuing medical treatment.

At the end of May 1948, Leriche left for Holland. Kunlin's patient was about to lose his leg so he agreed to Kunlin's proposal. The operation was performed on June 3, 1948. Instead of performing end-to-end anastomoses, Kunlin's proposal utilized an end-to-side technique, reasoning that collaterals could be preserved and the anastomoses would be easier. Within 3 weeks of the bypass, the patient's foot ulcer had healed.

Upon his return from Holland, Leriche was astonished that the procedure had been successful. Nevertheless, he encouraged Kunlin to continue his work. Kunlin's first patient underwent a contralateral bypass several months later, and survived for 1 year, until he suffered a stroke.

Kunlin's second patient was a 40-year-old man whose bypass remained patent for 8 years. Kunlin's third patient underwent bilateral femoral–popliteal

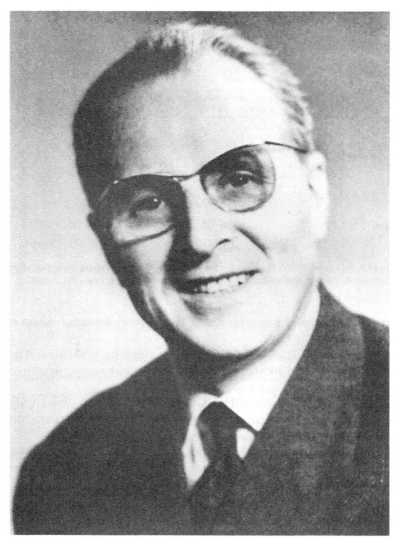

**Figure 19.1** Jean Kunlin (from Callow AD. Historical development of vascular grafts. In: Sawyer PN, Kaplitt MJ, eds. *Vascular Grafts*. New York: Appleton-Century-Crofts, 1978).

*Travail du Service de M. le Pr R. LERICHE*
*(Hôpital Américain de Paris et Collège de France)*

# Le traitement de l'ischémie artéritique par la greffe veineuse longue

**par J. KUNLIN**
(Paris)

**avec la collaboration**
**des Drs C. BITRY-BOÉLY, VOLNIÉ et BEAUDRY** (1)

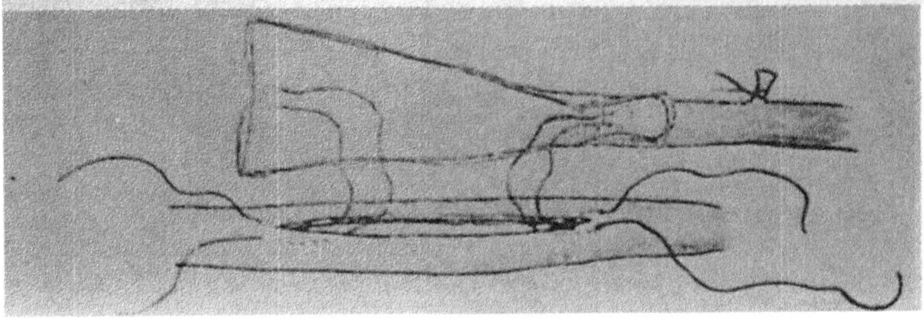

**Figure 19.2** Title page of Kunlin's account of the clinical use of venous bypass grafts (from Kunlin J. Le traitement de l'ischémie artéritique par la greffe veineuse longue. *Rev Chir* 1951; 70:206).

bypasses that remained patent for 28 and 25 years, with the aid of several additional procedures.

Kunlin (Figure 19.1) presented his first eight cases to the Academy of Sciences in November 1948, and his technique was soon adopted by surgeons around the world (Figure 19.2).

In 1962, Kunlin was appointed to the Hôpital Foch, in Paris, where he developed a department of vascular surgery. Soon after, he received the René Leriche award from the International Society of Surgery.

Kunlin retired 10 years later but continued his research activity in the Hôpital Foch Laboratory. In 1981, he was awarded the Vermeil Medal of Paris. Kunlin died in Paris on September 11, 1991, after a brief illness; he was 87.

## Bibliography

Cid Dos Santos J. From embolectomy to endarterectomy or the fall of a myth. *J Cardiovasc Surg* 1976; 17:113.

Kunlin J. Chirurge expérimentale: Sur l'auto-perfusuin cardio-encéphalique pendant l'exlusion de la circulation intra-cardiaque en vue de la chirurgie des cavités du coer. *CR Séances Acad Sci* 1948; 226:357.

Kunlin J. Exploration chirurgicale des cavités du coer gauche avec circulation coranoroencéphalique artificielle chez le chien. *CR Séances Acad Sci* 1948; 226:1863.

Kunlin J. Développement anéurysmatique après thrombo-endartériectomie de J Cid Dos Santos. *Mem Acad Chir* 1948; 74:553.

Kunlin J. Résultats de l'endartériectomie expérimentale. Etude histologique. *Mem Acad Chir* 1948; 74:557.

Kunlin J. Le traitement de l'ischémie artérique par la greffe veineuse longue. *Rev Chir* 1951; 70:206.

Kunlin J. Expériences de perfusions supra-diaphragmaiques et de circulation extra-corporéale totale chez le chien en vue de la chirurgie intra-cardiaque (au moyen d'un coer et d'un poumon artificiels). *Rev Chir* 1952; 237:2.

Kunlin J. Le rétablissement de la circulation veinuse par greffe en cas d'oblitération traumatique ou thrombophlébitique: greffe de 18 cm entre la veine saphéne interne et la veine iliaque externe. Thrombose après 3 semaines de perméabilité. *Mem Acad Chir* 1953; 79:109.

Kunlin J. *Die chirurgische Behandlung der obliterierenden Gefäß erkrankungen an den Extremitäten in Hans Hess. Die obliterierenden Gefäß erkrankungen.* Munich: Urban et Schwarzenberg, 1959.

Kunlin J. Introduction: Les étapes de la chirurgie vasculaire. In Dubost Ch. *Actuelle Chirurgie Cardiovasc* 1984; 3:1.

Kunlin J. Commentary. In Eklöf B, Gjöres JB, Thulesius O, Bergqvist D, eds. *Controversies in the Management of Venous Disorders.* London: Butterworths, 1990:289.

Kunlin J, Melon JM. Etude de la fibrillation et des moyens de defibrillation du coer chez le chien hiberné articicieliement (selon la méthode de Laborit) et soumis à l'arret circulatoire et à la ventriculotomie. *Presse Méd* 1956; 64:1063.

Kunlin J, Jaulmes C, Laborit H. Essais de chirurgie intracardiaque expérimentale exsangue sous hibernation articielle. *Mem Acad Chir* 1953; 79:664.

Leriche R. Des obliterations artérielles hautes (obliterations de la terminaison de l'aorte) comme causes des insuffisances circulatoires des membres inférieurs. *Bull Mem Soc Chir Paris* 1923; 49:1404.

Leriche R, Kunlin J. Possibilité de greffe veineuse de grande dimension (15 à 47 cm) dans les thromboses artérielles étendues: *CR Séances Acad Sci* 1948; 227:939.

May R. Der erste Bypass. *Actuelle Chir* 1970; 5:385.

May R. Die Geschichte des Venen-Bypass. *Angiologia* 1983; 5:139.

Porster E, Kunlin J, Schnoebein R, et al. Anastomose port-cave par greffe veineuse avec suture suspendue à des anneaux. *Mem Acad Chir* 1961; 87:797.

Testart J. Jean Kunlin (1904–1991). *Ann Vasc Surg* 1995; 9:1.

Woringer E, Kunlin J. Anastomose entre la carotide primitive et la carotide intra-cranienne ou la sylvienne par greffon selon la technique de la suture suspendue. *Neurochirurgie* 1963; 9:181.

# CHAPTER 20

# Charles Dubost

*Courage and grace is a formidable mixture. The only place to see it is the bullring.*

*(Marlene Dietrich)*

Charles Dubost was born in Saint-Gaultier, India, in October 1914. Soon after, his parents emigrated to France where his father owned a pharmacy in the Latin quarter of Paris. Dubost's decision to become a surgeon was made at the age of 10, when he had a severe case of appendicitis. He felt as if his surgeon had snatched him from the jaws of death, and he vowed to devote his life to comfort and heal others.

Dubost completed his humanities at Henri IV and Louis-le-Grand. He began his medical studies as an extern of the Paris hospitals in 1934. Four years later he began his internship. His surgical training was concentrated primarily in general and gastrointestinal surgery, with some urologic and pediatric surgery. All of Dubost's teachers noted his exceptional intelligence and dexterity.

Dubost's training was interrupted by World War II. He served as a lieutenant-doctor of a fortress artillery unit. After the liberation of France, Dubost was assigned to a mobile surgical group. At Clermont de l'Oise, he performed major operations under difficult conditions and was awarded the War Cross for his bravery.

After the war, Dubost's career was determined by two of the most renowned surgeons in Paris: François de Gaudart d'Allaines and Henri Mondor. de Gaudart d'Allaines knew Dubost as an extern. He offered him an internship on his own service, and Dubost soon became his first assistant.

In 1946, Dubost was named assistant-surgeon of hospitals in Paris. The general surgery service at Broussais Hospital, where Henri Mondor was the chief of surgery, became renowned because of Dubost's work in esophageal, gastric, and colorectal surgery.

In 1947, de Gaudart d'Allaines invited Alfred Blalock and Henry Bahnson to Paris, where they demonstrated their treatment of "blue" children. Dubost was impressed by the thoughtfulness and skill of these surgeons from Baltimore, and he resolved to devote himself to the nascent field of cardiac surgery. de Gaudart d'Allaines supported Dubost and reserved several beds on his service for the treatment of blue children. He also placed an animal laboratory at Dubost's disposal.

In 1949, Dubost became surgeon of hospitals in Paris (Figure 20.1). A year later, he resected a saccular aneurysm of the descending aorta.

On March 29, 1951, Dubost became the first surgeon to resect an abdominal aortic aneurysm and replace it with a homograft (Figure 20.2). His patient was a 50-year-old man, and the operation was performed via a left thoracoabdominal

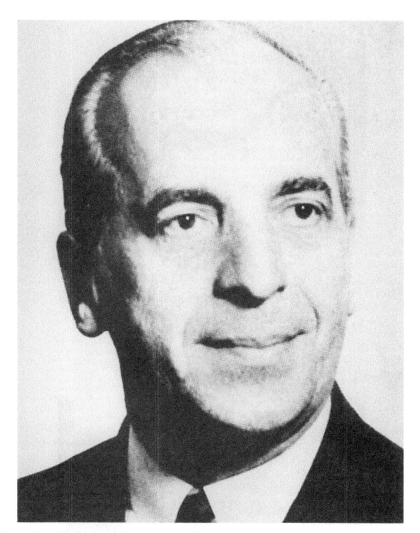

**Figure 20.1** Charles Dubost (from Dubost C. First successful resection of an aneurysm of an abdominal aorta with restoration of the continuity by a human arterial graft. *World J Surg* 1982; 6:256).

incision. A 15-cm homograft, taken from the thoracic aorta of a 20-year-old woman who had died 3 weeks earlier, was anastomosed to the aorta and right common iliac artery. An endarterectomy of the occluded left common iliac artery was performed before its anastomosis to the homograft. The patient survived for 8 years, succumbing to a myocardial infarction at his home in Brittany. The report of this operation rocked the surgical world and inspired surgeons throughout Europe and the United States. Several years later, Michael DeBakey performed a similar operation with a prosthesis and coined it: "Dubost's operation."

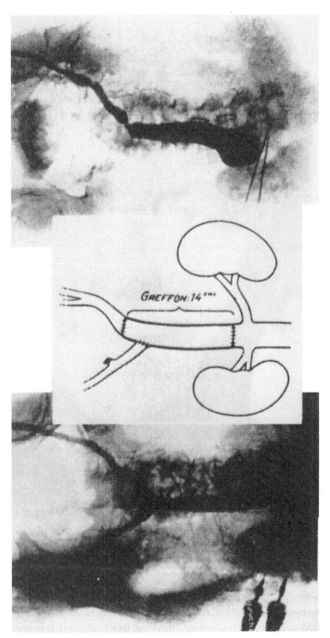

**Figure 20.2** Pre- and postoperative angiograms, and illustration of the first aneurysm resection with replacement by an arterial homograft (from Dubost C. Resection of an aneurysm of the abdominal aorta: Reestablishment of the continuity by a preserved human arterial graft, with results after five months. *Arch Surg* 1952; 64:405).

In 1951, Dubost also attempted the first renal transplant in Europe. The donor probably did not sign a surgical consent form, because he was a recently guillotined criminal from la Santé. Without the means to prevent rejection, however, the graft failed. Dubost was devastated and never attempted the procedure again.

Dubost continued to devote much of his time to cardiac surgery in the animal laboratory and in 1953 his efforts were rewarded when René Savage offered him a position in the new thoracic surgery center of Marie-Lannelongue. Dubost organized a 12-bed cardiac surgery unit and continued his laboratory research.

In 1955, Dubost passed the aggregation examination and became professor of surgery. That year he also became the first European to use a heart–lung machine during repair of a ventricular septal defect in a 6-year-old. Four years later, Dubost and Gérard Guiot used hypothermic circulatory arrest to successfully excise a large cerebral angioma. This was another "first in the world" for Dubost. Dubost eventually used this technique in more than 200 operations to correct tetralogy of Fallot, pulmonary stenosis, atrial–ventricular malformations, and cardiac septal defects.

In 1963, Dubost succeeded de Gaudart d'Allaines at Broussais. He was appointed chairman of cardiovascular surgery and chief of the new Leriche service. From this position, he encouraged Alain Carpentier to develop a prosthetic heart valve. In 1968, Carpentier implanted the first valve prosthesis in a human, at Broussais. That same year, Dubost also became the first European surgeon to perform cardiac transplantation. His patient, Father Damien Boulogne, survived for 16 months, during which he and Dubost became close friends. In fact, the only photograph in Dubost's office was of Boulogne. When asked why only that photo, Dubost replied, "He showed me what courage is."

In 1971, Dubost performed the first decortication procedure for endocarditis. During his career of four decades, Dubost oversaw more than 15 000 open-heart procedures. He performed more than 800 repairs of coarctations and continued Jean Kunlin's work with lower extremity revascularization. Patients throughout Europe flocked to Broussais and Marie-Lannelongue because of his reputation.

Between 1969 and 1975, Dubost was elected Honorary Fellow of the Society of Thoracic Surgeons, of the American College of Surgeons, and of the American Surgical Association. In 1975, he was elected to the Academy of Sciences, and 3 years later he was elected to the Academy of Medicine.

Dubost retired in 1982. During his last decade, he read, enjoyed classical music, and entertained many of the friends and students he had known throughout his career. Dubost died at Saint-Michel Hospital in 1991.

In his eulogy to Dubost, Maurice Mercadier best described the respect and affection that shone on him:

> He incised, he cleaved, dissected, resectioned and reconstituted the tissues or the organs without a hitch, without haste, and without a wasted gesture. The intervention he realized took place like a harmonious ballet of elegant movements . . . To help him was a joy, and all help had the exalted feeling of participating in a magic ritual with happy

results. Thus is explained the admiring affection of his students and his staff, of his technicians and his nurses, whom I thank for having come en masse to pay him homage.

## Bibliography

Binet JP. Nécrologie Charles Dubost. *Chirurgie* 1991; 517:107.

Blondeau P. Nécrologie Charles Dubost. *Arch Mal Coeur* 1992; 85:483.

Dubost C. Resection of an aneurysm of the abdominal aorta. *Arch Surg* 1952; 64:405.

Dubost C. First successful resection of an aneurysm of the abdominal aorta with restoration of the continuity by a human arterial graft. *World J Surg* 1982; 6:256.

Mercadier M. Éloge de Charles Dubost. *Bull Acad Natl Med* 1991;175:1005.

# CHAPTER 21

# Jacques Oudot

*A few hours' mountain climbing turns a rogue and a saint into two roughly equal creatures.*
*Weariness is the shortest path to equality and fraternity – and liberty is finally added by sleep.*

*(Friedrich Nietzsch)*

Jacques Oudot was born in Dammarie-les-Lys in 1913. Little has been written about his childhood, but it is known that he did not consider a career in medicine until his third decade of life. Oudot began his career in chemistry and pharmacy, and actually began a pharmacy residency before evincing an interest in surgery.

In 1946, Oudot wrote his thesis on vasodilatation. He remained interested in blood vessels and began research in vascular surgery during the next few years.

By 1950, Oudot was assistant surgeon at the Paris hospitals (Figure 21.1). Most of his time was spent at the animal experimental center of the Anatomy Laboratory, rue du Fer à Moulin. Oudot's experimental work there was divided into three parts. The initial stage involved creation of a dog model for chronic aortic occlusion. Early attempts with an active thrombin called topostasine were unsuccessful because of the rapidity with which thrombosis occurred. Next, Oudot wrapped the aortic trifurcation (the canine hypogastric arteries originate in a common trunk from the aorta) with Cellophane and achieved success in three animals. These dogs had hind limb claudication without paraplegia.

The second phase of Oudot's work concentrated on the effects of transient aortic clamping on the kidneys, lungs, and carotid and femoral artery pressures. He ultimately learned that animals could tolerate transient acute aortic occlusion.

Finally, Oudot tested many solutions for homograft preservation. He harvested grafts from animals humanely sacrificed at a local pound and placed them in a modified Tyrode's solution. The grafts were then refrigerated for several days to 4 weeks. Oudot found that the grafts remained grossly normal and were strong enough to hold sutures.

In 1950, Oudot and Jean Natali operated on 20 dogs. Their initial mortality rate was 100 percent; however, by October they had achieved survival in eight of 10 animals. They attributed their improved results to greater experience, less traumatic clamps, and the procurement of finer needles. Their experiments were continued through 1951, and one dog eventually lived for 10 years.

On November 14, 1950, Oudot operated on a 51-year-old woman with aortic occlusion and nonhealing ulcers of the left leg. A retroperitoneal approach was used and, as might have been predicted, Oudot had considerable difficulty with

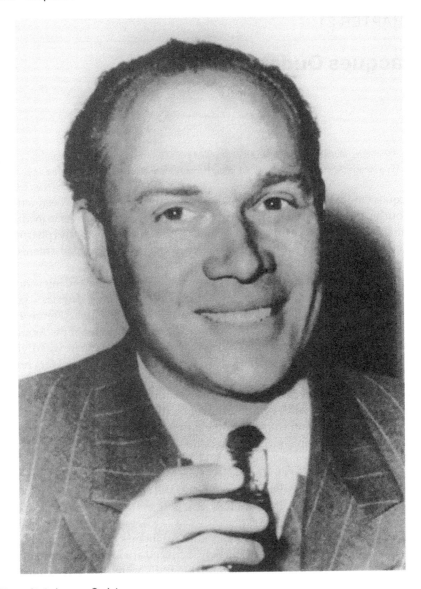

**Figure 21.1** Jacques Oudot.

the right iliac anastomosis. The left iliac anastomosis was uncomplicated. Oudot's patient did well postoperatively, but the right femoral pulse was absent. On May 8, 1951, Oudot performed the first crossover bypass by inserting a graft between her two external iliac arteries. These two procedures were also remarkable because they defied the prediction of René Leriche, who favored lumbar sympathectomy over direct vascular reconstruction. The patient survived until 1954. Her autopsy revealed thrombosis of the homograft.

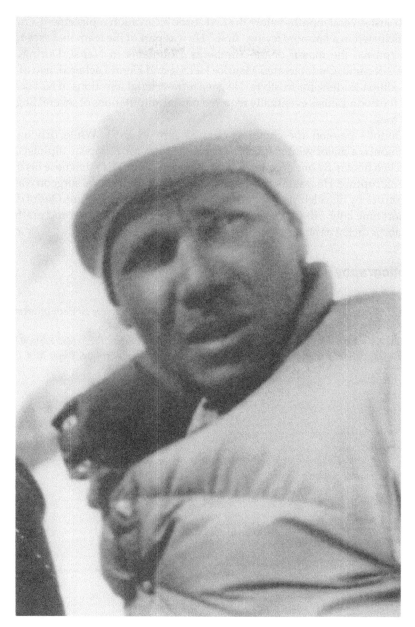

**Figure 21.2** Jacques Oudot's other passion: mountain climbing.

The second aortic bifurcation graft was performed on May 16, 1951. The patient made an uneventful recovery. During the next 2 years, Oudot operated on 11 additional patients. Four died and seven survived with satisfactory results.

Oudot had a passion other than surgery: mountain climbing (Figure 21.2). In

1950, just several months before the first aortic bifurcation replacement, Oudot participated in a far more trying "first." He was part of the team that ascended Annapurna, the massif of the Himalaya Mountains in Nepal. During the 26 502-ft climb, Oudot treated Maurice Herzog and Henri Lachenal, two of the expedition leaders, for frostbite. He gave intra-arterial injections of Novocain, and the two alpinists eventually required partial amputations of several fingers and toes.

Oudot's passion for climbing claimed him in 1953. While driving to Chamonix, a major winter sports resort and Mecca for European alpinists, he wrecked his car. By one account, Oudot lived long enough to diagnose his own splenic rupture. He was taken to a small hospital where the local surgeon was so awestruck by his celebrity patient that he dared not operate on him. Oudot died a short time later. His promising work on kidney transplantation and grafts of the aortic arch was never published.

## Bibliography

Ichac M, Herzog M. *Regards vers l'Annapurna*. Paris: B. Arthaud, 1951.

Natali J. Hommage à Jacques Oudot pour le 50 anniversaire de la première greffe de bifurcation aortique. *Chirurgie* 1999; 124:448.

Oudot J. Observations physiologiques et cliniques en haute montagne. *Presse Med* 1951; 59:227.

Oudot J. La greffe vasculaire dans les thromboses du carrefour aortique. *Presse Med* 1951; 59:234.

# PART 7

**Endovascular surgery**

# CHAPTER 22

# Charles Dotter: interventional radiologist

*Innovation violates tradition – attacks it in public and steals from it in private.*

(Mason Cooley)

Charles Dotter was born in Boston, Massachusetts, on June 14, 1920. His family moved to Freeport, Long Island, when Dotter was an infant. Dotter's father was a successful stock trader and his mother was an aspiring actress.

Dotter attended grammar school, where he skipped a grade, and high school in Freeport and was an excellent student. Dotter was always small for his age and eschewed competitive sports. He turned to mountain climbing as an outlet for his boundless energy and displayed an early mechanical aptitude. Dotter derived great satisfaction from working with tools and adopted his own sketch of a plumber's tools to symbolize his interest (Figure 22.1). Dotter rarely observed a mechanical device or machine without contemplating other uses for it.

After graduation from high school in Freeport, Dotter attended Duke University. He received a bachelor of arts degree in 1941. Dotter returned to New York to attend medical school at Cornell, where he met his future wife, Pamela Battie. She was a head nurse at New York Hospital and they were married in 1944. Dotter completed his internship at the United States Naval Hospital in St. Albans, New York, and his radiology residency at New York Hospital.

In 1950, Dotter became a full-time member of the Cornell University Medical College faculty. That year he developed an automatic x-ray roll-film magazine capable of producing two images per second. This became the prototype for the grid-controlled x-ray tube. Two years later, Dotter was appointed Professor and Chairman of the Department of Radiology at the University of Oregon Medical School. At age 32, he was the youngest person to become chairman of a radiology department in a major American medical school. He held the position for 32 years, during which he published over 300 manuscripts, produced three scientific training films, and created a new medical specialty: interventional radiology.

By the early 1960s, Dotter had written more than 100 articles, many dealing with the diagnosis of acquired and congenital cardiac lesions, developing new contrast media, and describing new ways to visualize the peripheral vascular system. Dotter realized, however, that the key to a new medical specialty based upon endovascular interventions was the manufacture of catheters of various shapes and sizes. Dotter and his laboratory technicians used blow torches to fabricate catheters from speedometer cables, guitar strings, and vinyl cable insulation. Dotter lacked a reliable means of mass production of wires and catheters.

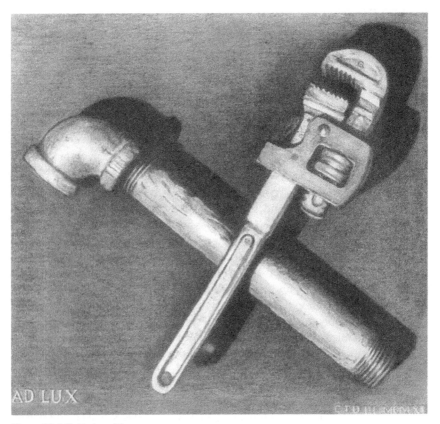

**Figure 22.1** Dotter's emblem.

Enter Bill Cook. In 1963, Dotter met Cook at the Radiologic Society of North America meeting in Chicago. Cook later recalled their meeting:

> We discussed wire guide and catheter manufacture and what he thought the future would be for angiography. He became excited when he talked of his work, and yes, we discussed angioplasty. He hauled out the picture of his plumber's wrenches that we've all looked at so many times. Once started, his mind went nonstop.

Cook visited Dotter at his lab in Oregon and viewed his sketches of telescopic catheters. From these, the first Dotter dilatation set was produced, setting the stage for the first percutaneous transluminal angioplasty. Two more important events preceded this.

In 1963, Dotter conducted a postmortem study of the feasibility of coronary radiography and endarterectomy. He noted that forceful intraluminal hydraulic injections through stenotic areas led to an increase in flow across these lesions. Dotter reasoned that local catheter dilatation might have therapeutic value in cases of lower extremity ischemia due to focal stenoses. He believed the risk of distal embolization was slight and that percutaneous transluminal dilatation could be a simple and valuable technique.

The second important event in 1963 was an accident. During an abdominal aortogram in a patient with renal artery stenosis, Dotter inadvertently recanalized an occluded right iliac artery. He immediately pondered the possibilities had a balloon been attached to the catheter.

Laura Shaw was 82 years old when she was admitted to the University of Oregon Hospital with gangrene and rest pain of the left foot. All of her physicians had recommended an amputation, including her vascular surgeon. When Shaw refused surgery, her vascular surgeon asked Dotter to see her. An angiogram revealed a focal stenosis of the superficial femoral artery and Dotter realized he had the ideal lesion with which to test his dilating catheter (Figure 22.2). On January 16, 1964, Dotter performed the first percutaneous transluminal angioplasty. The procedure went well and Shaw's foot became hyperemic. Her rest pain disappeared and within a few months her foot was healed. An angiogram performed 3 weeks later demonstrated a patent angioplasty; interventional radiology was born. Laura Shaw died of

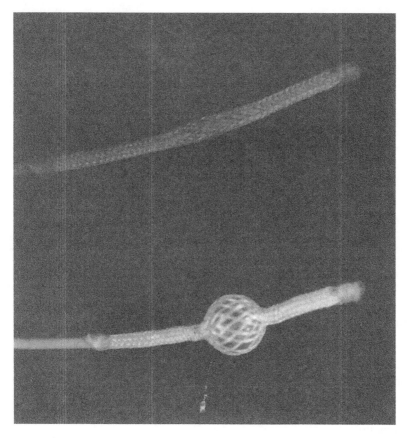

**Figure 22.2** Original Dotter dilating catheter (courtesy of Mrs. Enid Ruble).

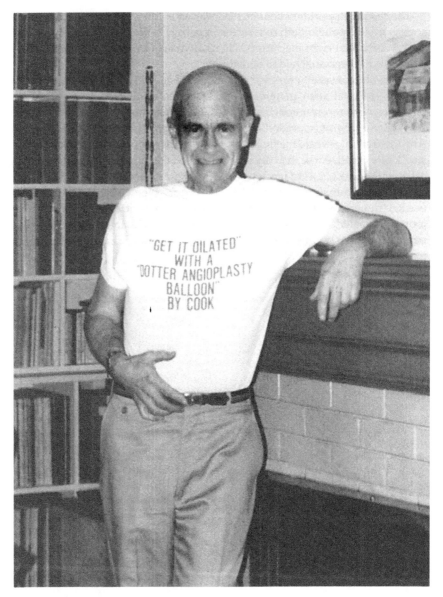

**Figure 22.3** Charles Dotter (courtesy of Mrs. Enid Ruble).

congestive heart failure nearly 3 years later, "still walking on my own two feet." Later in the year, Dotter reported good results with 15 angioplasties in 11 lower extremities (Figure 22.3). He was prescient of other applications for this new technique:

If its use in femoral disease can be taken as an indication severe proximal narrowing of the coronary artery will be amenable to a manually guided dilator inserted via aortotomy or via the brachial artery by the Sones technic. Proximal stenosis of the renal, carotid, and vertebral arteries appears suitable for transvascular treatment. . . . It seems reasonable to expect that the transluminal technique for recanalization will extend the scope of treatment beyond the limits of present-day surgery.

Dotter's powerful innovation initially received more interest in Europe than the United States, owing to the excellent results obtained in preliminary trials of this technique abroad. European radiologists referred to percutaneous transluminal angioplasty as "Dottering" (Figure 22.4).

Dotter pioneered other areas of interventional radiology. He developed catheters with which to retrieve foreign bodies from the vascular and gastrointestinal systems. In 1972, he described a new method for control of acute gastrointestinal bleeding: selective arterial embolization. Dotter described the use of cyanoacrylate for therapeutic vascular occlusion and he was the first to employ intra-arterial fibrinolytic agents. The original description of intravascular stents was also Dotter's.

Despite the appearance of enlarged lymph nodes in his axilla in 1967, Dotter continued his practice and research, and his outdoor pursuits (Figure 22.5). Until he began suffering night sweats 2 years later, Dotter brooked no interruption of his work schedule. A biopsy revealed Hodgkin's disease, and Dotter

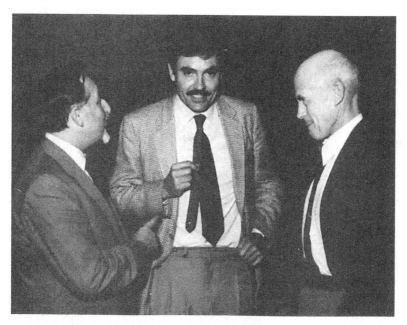

**Figure 22.4** Pioneers of interventional radiology: Egerhardt Zeitler (left), Andreas Gruentzig (center), and Charles Dotter (right) (courtesy of Mrs. Enid Ruble).

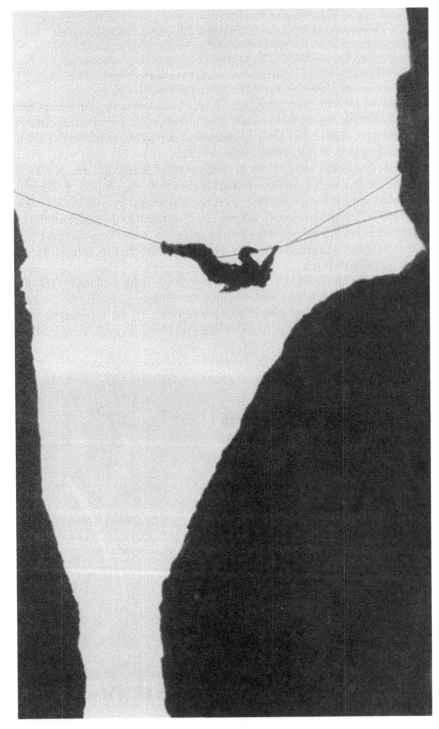

**Figure 22.5** Charles Dotter rock climbing in central Oregon in 1968 (reproduced with permission from Friedman SG. Charles Dotter: Interventional radiologist. *Radiology* 1989; 172:921).

simply arranged his radiation therapy around his clinical responsibilities. He responded well to therapy, worked throughout, and celebrated by climbing the Matterhorn, without a guide, in 1970. Dotter eventually scaled all 67 peaks exceeding 14 000 feet in the continental United States. He also continued his interest in painting, photography, classical music, and hiking with his wife and their three children. Dotter suffered a recurrence of Hodgkin's disease in 1976, and worked throughout a second course of radiation therapy.

Health problems continued to plague Dotter, and his frenetic daily schedule did not help. In 1979, while backpacking in the Wallowa mountains in eastern Oregon, he experienced exertional dyspnea. In April 1979, Dotter underwent a quadruple coronary bypass, from which he made a slow recovery. In February 1980, Dotter survived surgery for a perforated duodenal ulcer and was soon back to teaching, practice, and the outdoors.

Dotter's love of nature, mechanical aptitude, and his simple approach to problems are all displayed in a letter he wrote to a friend in 1982. Dotter had long been interested in the plight of California's condors and he had visited Santa Barbara on several occasions to observe these birds. Several condor eggs had been lost by rolling off the edge of a particular cliff where the birds nested. Dotter conceived a solution and immediately wrote and telephoned the authorities to effect it (Figure 22.6).

Dotter received many awards during his career, including gold medals from the Radiologic Society of North America, the Chicago Medical Society, and the Chicago Radiological Society, in 1981. He received an American College of

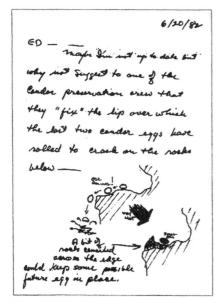
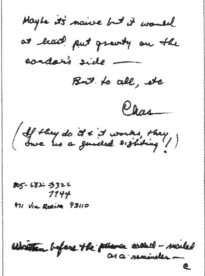

**Figure 22.6** Dotter's solution to lost condor eggs (reproduced with permission from Friedman SG. Charles Dotter: Interventional radiologist. *Radiology* 1989; 172:921).

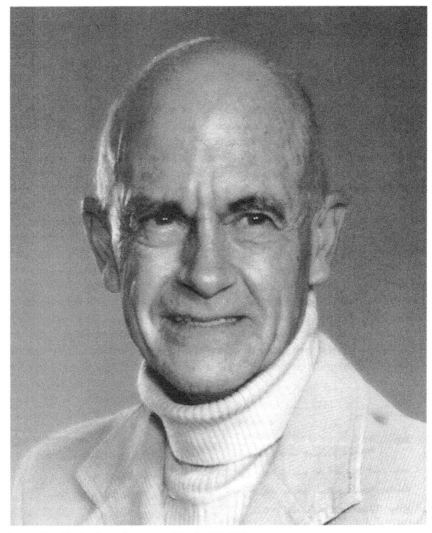

**Figure 22.7** Charles Dotter (courtesy of Mrs. Enid Ruble).

Radiology gold medal 2 years later. The greatest indication of the regard for Dotter by his peers was his nomination, by an editor of Year Book Medical Publishers, to receive the Nobel Prize in Medicine in 1978 (Figure 22.7).

Dotter's health failed again in 1983, when he developed recurrent angina and dyspnea on exertion. In August 1983, he underwent repeat coronary bypass, and mitral valve replacement. The operation lasted 12 hours, and not even Dotter could fully recover from such an ordeal. He was unable to resume work and his condition slowly deteriorated. During the ensuing months, Dotter was cared

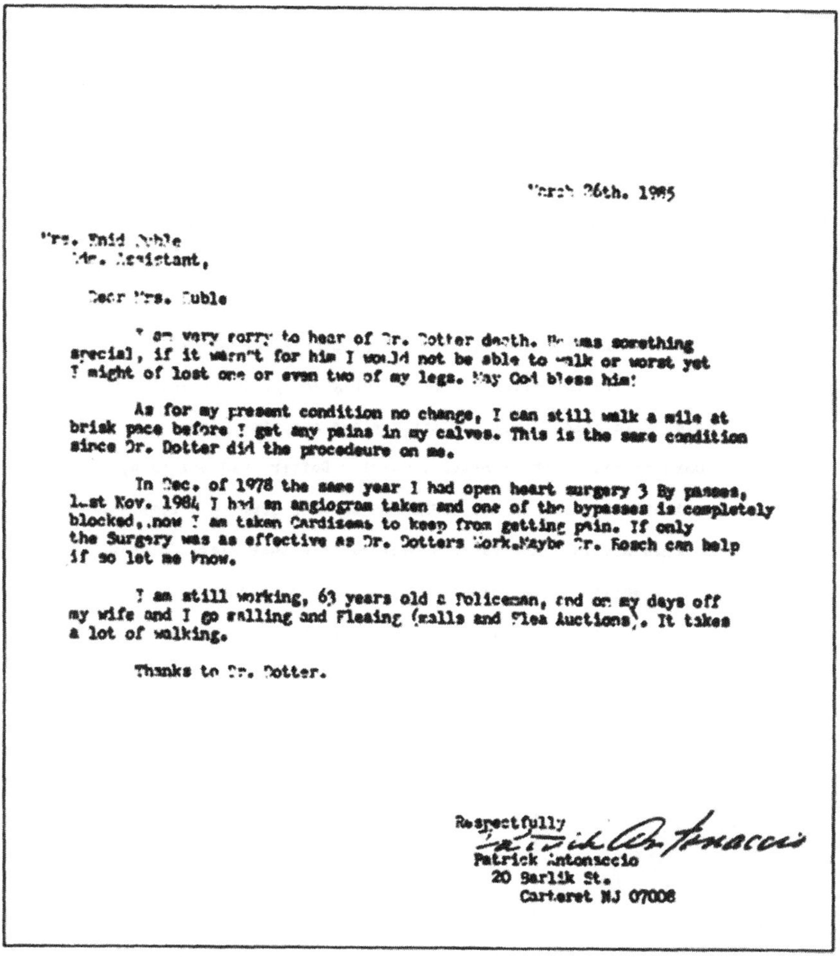

> ‛arc‛ 26th. 1985
>
> ''rs. Enid Noble
>   Mr. Assistant,
>
>   Dear Mrs. Nuble
>
>       I am very sorry to hear of Dr. Dotter death. He was something
>   special, if it warn't for him I would not be able to walk or worst yet
>   I might of lost one or even two of my legs. May God bless him!
>
>       As for my present condition no change, I can still walk a mile at
>   brisk pace before I get any pains in my calves. This is the same condition
>   since Dr. Dotter did the procedeure on me.
>
>       In Dec. of 1978 the same year I had open heart surgery 3 By passes,
>   Last Nov. 1984 I had an angiogram taken and one of the bypasses is completely
>   blocked, now I am taken Cardizem to keep from getting pain. If only
>   the Surgery was as effective as Dr. Dotters Work. Maybe Dr. Rosch can help
>   if so let me know.
>
>       I am still working, 63 years old a Policeman, and on my days off
>   my wife and I go salling and Fleaing (malls and Flea Auctions). It takes
>   a lot of walking.
>
>       Thanks to Dr. Dotter.
>
>                                           Respectfully
>                                           Patrick Antonaccio
>                                           20 Sarlik St.
>                                           Carteret NJ 07008

**Figure 22.8** Letter of sympathy from a patient who had undergone bilateral iliac dilations (reproduced with permission from Friedman SG. Charles Dotter: Interventional radiologist. *Radiology* 1989; 172:921).

for at home by his wife and daughter, both nurses. In 1985, a tragic year for the field of radiology, Dotter was readmitted to the hospital for respiratory failure, from which he died on February 15. In that year, three other preeminent interventional radiologists also died: Melvin Judkins, F. Mason Sones, Jr., and Andreas Gruentzig.

Dotter's death evoked an outpouring of praise and sorrow from patients and physicians around the world (Figures 22.8 and 22.9). Dotter changed the practice of medicine and had an indelible impact upon those who met him. Millions of patients owe their lives and limbs to Dotter's innovations. Dr. Leonard Laser, then president of the Oregon Health Sciences University, summarized Dotter's life best:

Dear Dotters!

Dear Pamela Dotter and your children!

We've learnt about the decease of the great contemporary scientist Charles Dotter with deep sorrow. he was a man of extraordinary abilities and talent. As a researcher he won the recognition all over the world. Our scientists revere the memory of the big friend of the Soviet people. My personal encounter with Ch.Dotter impressed me greatly. I remember our scientific discussions, creative plans and simply personal human contact. Unfortunately, Charles Dotter had not an opportunity to come to the USSR. And in this country a symposium on endovascular interference will be held this year. Charles Dotter was to be an honour guest at this symposium."

We will always remember Ch.Dotter as a founder of the new trend in clinical medicine. Charles Dotter was an outstanding scientist, wonderful person and a true friend.

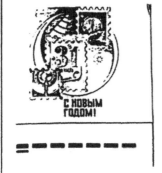

With the best regards

Prof. I.Rabkin

119435 USSR, Moscow,
Abrikosovsky 2, National
Research Center of Surgery,
Prof. J. Rabkin

**Figure 22.9** Letter of sympathy from Dr. I. Rabkin of the Soviet Union (reproduced with permission from Friedman SG. Charles Dotter: Interventional radiologist. *Radiology* 1989; 172:921).

Rarely in the course of a medical career is an individual granted the opportunity to alter forever the course of medicine for human good. Charles Dotter was one of those happy few.

## Bibliography

Bilbao MK, Krippaehne WW, Dotter CT. Catheter retrieval of foreign body from the gastrointestinal tract. *AJR* 1971; 111:473.

Dotter CT. Urokon sodium 50%, hypaque 50%, renograffin 59.7% for intravenous urography: experimental, clinical comparison. *Radiologica* 1956; 7:12.

Dotter CT. Left ventricular and systemic arterial catheterization: a simple percutaneous method using a spring guide. *Am J Roentgenol* 1960; 83:969.

Dotter CT. Transluminally placed coil-spring endarterial tube grafts: long term patency in canine popliteal artery. *Invest Radiol* 1969; 4:329.

Dotter CT, Judkins MP. Transluminal treatment of arteriosclerotic obstuction. Description of a new technic and a preliminary report of its application. *Circulation* 1964; 30:654.

Dotter CT, Steinberg I. The diagnosis of congenital aneurysm of the pulmonary artery. *N Engl J Med* 1949; 240:51.

Dotter CT, Steinberg I. Advances in angiocardiography. *Med Clin North Am* 1950; 34:745.

Dotter CT, Roesch J, Bilbao MK. Transluminal extraction of catheter and guide fragments from the heart and great vessels: 29 collected cases. *Am J Roentgenol* 1971; 111:467.

Dotter CT, Goldman ML, Roesch, J. Instant selective arterial occlusion with isobutyl 2-cyanoacrylate. *Radiology* 1975; 114:227.

Fogarty TJ, Chin A, Shoor PM, *et al*. Adjunctive intraoperative arterial dilatation. Simplified instrumentation technique. *Arch Surg* 1981; 116:1391.

Greenfield AJ. Femoral, popliteal and tibial arteries: percutaneous transluminal angioplasty. *Am J Roentgenol* 1980; 135:928.

Gruentzig AR. Results from coronary angioplasty and implications for the future. *Am Heart J* 1982; 103:779.

Gruentzig AR, Hopff H. Perkutaene rekanalisation chronischer arterieller verschluess mit einem neuen dilatationskatheter. *Dtsch Med Wschr* 1974; 99:2502.

Gruentzig AR, Kumpe DA. Technique of percutaneous transluminal angioplasty with the Gruentzig balloon catheter. *Am J Roentgenol* 1979; 132:547.

Gruentzig AR, Myler RK, Hanna ES, *et al*. Coronary transluminal angioplasty. (abstract) *Circulation* 1977; 56(Suppl II):319.

Johnston KW, Rae M, Hogg-Johnston SA, *et al*. 5-year results of a prospective study of percutaneous transluminal angioplasty. *Ann Surg* 1987; 206:403.

Katzen BT, Change J, Knox G. Percutaneous transluminal angioplasty with the Gruentzig balloon catheter. *Arch Surg* 1979; 114:1389.

Niles NR, Dotter CT. Coronary radiography and endarterectomy. Postmortem study of feasibility of surgery. *Circulation* 1963; 28:190.

Porstmann W. Ein neuer korsett-ballonkatheter zur transluminalen rekanalisation nach Dotter unter besonderer beruecksichtigung von obliterationen an den beckenarterien. *Radiol Diagn* 1973; 14:239.

Porstmann W, Wierny L. Intravasale rekanalisation inoperabler arterieller obliterationen. *Zentralbl Chir* 1967; 92:1586.

Roesch J, Dotter CT, Brown MJ. Selective arterial embolization: a new method for control of acute gastrointestinal bleeding. *Radiology* 1972; 102:303.

Sanborn TA, Greenfield AJ, Guben JK, *et al*. Human percutaneous and intraoperative laser thermal angioplasty – Initial clinical results as an adjunct to balloon angioplasty. *J Vasc Surg* 1987; 5:83.

Schwarten DE. Transluminal angioplasty of renal artery stenosis: 70 experiences. *Am J Roentgenol* 1980; 135:969.

Zeitler E, Muller R. Erste ergebnisse mit der katheter – rekanalisation nach Dotter bei arterieller verschlusskrankheit. *Roefo* 1969; 111:345.

# CHAPTER 23

# Thomas Fogarty

*Wine comes in at the mouth*
*And love comes in at the eye;*
*That's all we shall know for truth*
*Before we grow old and die.*

*(William Butler Yeats)*

Thomas Fogarty was born in Cincinnati, Ohio, on February 25, 1934. He attended Catholic grade school and was an average student. When Fogarty was 10 years old his father died, forcing him to begin delivering newspapers and mowing lawns to help make ends meet. In the eighth grade, Fogarty began working in the central supply department of Good Samaritan Hospital. Fogarty remained at Good Samaritan during his attendance at Roger Bacon High School, eventually becoming a scrub technician. It was in this role that he met Dr. Jack Cranley, an eminent vascular surgeon of that time.

As a teenager, Fogarty preferred boxing and riding motorcycles to studying. One of his friends owned a Cushman motor scooter with a treacherous gearbox. When shifting from a high to low gear the scooter would accelerate wildly, often propelling the rear passenger into the street. Fogarty and his friend developed a centrifugal clutch to ease the transition between gears, and Cushman eventually adopted it as their own. At the age of 16, Fogarty learned the value of a patent the hard way (Figure 23.1).

Fogarty performed poorly in high school and had difficulty obtaining recommendations for college. His principal commented that it would be an enormous waste of money and effort for any college to accept him. Nevertheless, in 1952 Fogarty entered Xavier University under probation. Contrary to predictions, he did well and graduated with honors. While he was a premedical student, Fogarty worked nights and weekends for tuition money and self-support.

Following college graduation, Fogarty entered The University of Cincinnati College of Medicine where he continued to work with Cranley. During his high school years, while working as an operating room scrub technician, Fogarty had noticed that embolectomies were cumbersome procedures and they were often unsuccessful. They were performed using suction catheters, saline flushes, local removal via multiple arteriotomies, vein strippers, corkscrew devices, and milking with Esmarch bandages. The variety of techniques used underscored the absence of a reliable one. Fogarty surmised there should be a better way to perform embolectomies, but he had no time to develop alternative methods until he was in medical school. There he began tinkering with latex gloves and ureteral catheters in an effort to design an efficient clot-removal device.

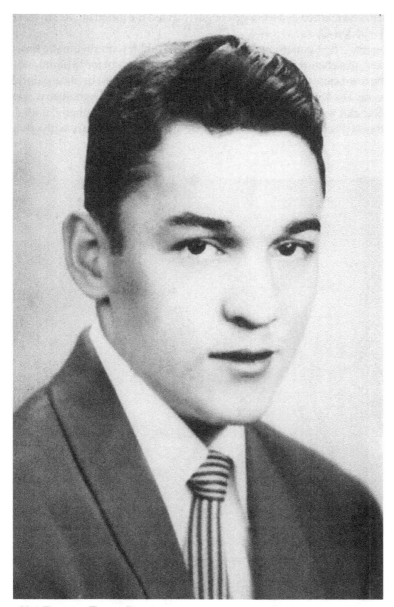

**Figure 23.1** The young Thomas Fogarty.

Fogarty graduated from medical school in 1960, and then completed a rotating internship at the University of Oregon Medical School. He returned to Cincinnati, where Cranley engaged him in a vascular fellowship for 1 year. It was during that year that Fogarty evaluated his new balloon embolectomy catheters. They were constructed from 6-French ureteral catheters and the fingertips of size 5 latex gloves that were attached using fly-tying techniques that

Fogarty had learned as a teenager. Fogarty tested the initial models in test tubes filled with Jell-O.

Fogarty's first patient was a 63-year-old woman with rheumatic heart disease and an ischemic left leg. Symptoms had been present for 18 hours and, during the few hours prior to Fogarty's examination, the foot became painful and insensate. The femoral pulse was absent and a diagnosis of embolism was made. The iliac clot was extracted with a Fogarty embolectomy catheter, under local anesthesia (Figure 23.2). The patient made an excellent recovery with salvage of

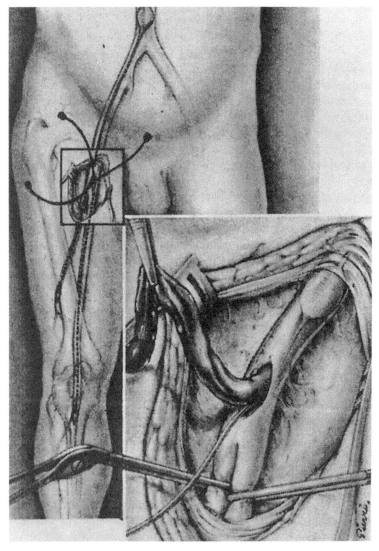

**Figure 23.2** Use of the Fogarty catheter (Fogarty TJ, Crauley JJ, Krause RJ, *et al*. A method for extraction of arterial emboli and thrombi. *Surg Gynecol Obstet* 1963; 116:241).

her limb. Dr. Jack Cranley, Fogarty's friend and mentor, performed this first surgery. By the end of that year, Fogarty recorded 11 additional successful cases of limb salvage with his balloon catheter. Despite this success, Fogarty was unable to find a manufacturer to invest in his novel device.

Fogarty returned to Oregon in 1962 to begin his surgical residency. Albert Starr MD, chief of cardiothoracic surgery, asked Lowell Edwards if he was interested in making balloon catheters. One year later, their mass production began. That year Fogarty also published "A Method for Extraction of Arterial Emboli and Thrombi" in "The Surgeon at Work" section of *Surgery, Gynecology & Obstetrics*. All would-be medical authors should be heartened by the fact that this manuscript was initially rejected by three other leading surgical journals. Fogarty summarized his early results:

> Admittedly our experience with this technique is not extensive, yet the ease and simplicity with which the artery can be cleared by this method has convinced us that it is distinctly superior to all others we have tried.

Upon his return to Oregon, Fogarty met Charles Dotter, who had recently developed an arterial dilating catheter. It was a remarkable coincidence that the authors of the first endovascular procedures worked at the same institution. Although Dotter provided Fogarty with some difficult cases as a result of unsuccessful dilations, Fogarty's superiors discouraged him from associating with Dotter because of his eccentric nature. One can only imagine the gifts to the medical field that might have resulted from the collaboration of these innovative men. Their partnership would have rivaled the collaboration of Carrel and Guthrie of a half-century earlier. Despite the admonishment of his peers, Fogarty constructed the first balloon catheters successfully used for iliac artery dilation by Dotter.

Following his third year of residency, Fogarty decided to take a year off to do research in cardiovascular physiology. He told Bert Dunphy of his desire to go to the University of Washington for this, whereupon Dunphy phoned a colleague, Dr. Andrew G. Morrow, at the NIH in Washington, DC, to make arrangements. After Fogarty explained that he meant the state of Washington, Dunphy replied: "You are going to the NIH in Washington, DC. It's a great opportunity and you will be back in two years."

Fogarty spent 1965–7 at the NIH, where he did clinical and basic science research. He also married Rosalee Brennan, whom he had met several years earlier at the University of Oregon, where she worked in the record room between college semesters. A year later, the first of their four children was born.

In 1967, Fogarty returned to the University of Oregon and finished his residency in general surgery, followed by completion of a cardiac surgery residency under Norman Shumway, MD, at Stanford University. Fogarty then entered private practice because, ironically, it afforded him more time for research than full-time academic practice. He continued his private practice at Stanford until 1978. In addition to continuing his research, Fogarty also began making wine as a hobby. By 1981, grape stomping was a serious avocation and, a decade later, the Thomas Fogarty Winery and Vineyards was making over ten thousand cases a year and distributing wine to states outside of California (Figure 23.3).

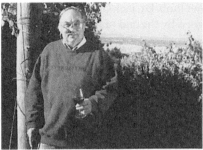

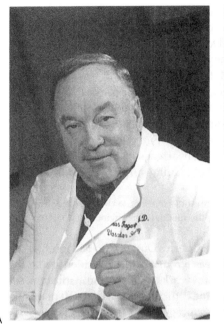

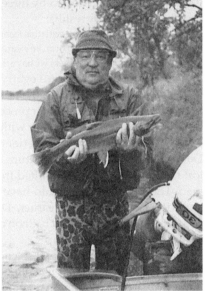

**Figure 23.3** (A–C) The three passions of Dr. Thomas Fogarty.

A

B

C

In 1980, Fogarty became Director of Cardiovascular Surgery at Sequoia Hospital in Redwood City, California. That same year he was named "Inventor of the Year" by the San Francisco Patent and Trademark Association. Fogarty remained at Sequoia until 1993, when he returned to Stanford University as Professor of Surgery. He maintains a clinical appointment there and limits his practice to endovascular surgery.

The careers of academic surgeons are customarily judged by their contributions to the literature. Based upon the sum of the medical companies founded (more than 40), plus the number of patents awarded in surgical instrumentation (more than 100), Fogarty's accomplishments established a new standard for assessing productivity. In addition to more than 200 publications, he founded AneuRx, Inc. (Medtronic AVE); Novare, Inc.; Cardiovascular Imaging Systems, Inc.; Bacchus Vascular, Inc.; Vascular Architects, Inc., and many other companies.

Other honors Fogarty garnered include The Lemelson–MIT $500,000 Prize for Invention and Innovation (2000), The Laufman–Greatbach Prize from the Association for the Advancement of Medical Instrumentation (2000), The International Society Award for Excellence in Endovascular Innovation bestowed by the International Society of Endovascular Specialists (2001), and the prestigious Jacobson Innovation Award of the American College of Surgeons (2001).

In December 2001, Fogarty received the ultimate recognition for his innovations: induction into The National Inventor's Hall of Fame.

## Bibliography

Dale WA. Endovascular suction catheters. *J Thorac Cardiovasc Surg* 1962; 44:557.

Dale WA, Johnson G, DeWeese JA, eds. *Band of Brothers*. Thomas James Fogarty. Appleton Communications, 1992.

Dotter C. Transluminal angioplasty: a long view. *Radiology* 1980; 135:561.

Fogarty TJ, Cranley JJ, Krause RJ, *et al*. A method for extraction of arterial emboli and thrombi. *Surg Gynecol Obstet* 1963; 116:241.

Green RM, DeWeese JA, Rob CG. Arterial embolectomy before and after the Fogarty catheter. *Surgery* 1975; 77:24.

Keeley JL. Saddle embolus of the aorta, report of successful embolectomy. *Ann Surg* 1948; 128:257.

Keeley JL, Rooney JA. Retrograde milking: An adjunct in technic of embolectomy. *Ann Surg* 1951; 134:1022.

Key E. Embolectomy in the treatment of circulatory disturbances in the extremities. *Surg Gynecol Obstet* 1923; 36:309.

Krause RJ, Cranley JJ. Management of peripheral arterial embolism. *Ohio St Med J* 1958; 54:485.

Krause RJ, Cranley JJ, Baylon LM, *et al*. Recent advancements in the treatment of peripheral arterial embolism. *Arch Surg* 1959; 79:285.

Lerman J, Miller FR, Lund CC. Arterial embolism and embolectomy. *JAMA* 1930; 94:1128.

Shaw RS. A method for the removal of the adherent distal thrombus. *Surg Gynecol Obstet* 1960; 110:255.

Softky, M. Cutting edge. *Money & Business* 1996; July 24:25.

*Surgical innovator wins $500,000 Lemelson–MIT Prize*. MIT Sloan School of Management Program 2000; 4: Summer.

# CHAPTER 24

# Juan Parodi

*The advancement of the arts, from year to year, taxes our credulity and seems to pre-sage the arrival of that period when human improvement must end.*

*(Henry L. Ellsworth, 1843, Commissioner of Patents)*

Juan Parodi was born on August 16, 1942, in Buenos Aires, Argentina. His mother was a teacher; his father managed a cattle ranch. Parodi was the third of four sons. Because his family lived in an area where many English companies were situated, Parodi attended an English school for the first 4 years of his education. He then attended a private school until the age of 12.

Parodi was a poor student and preferred shooting air rifles to studying. He spent countless hours riding horses, conducting mock warfare with his friends, and delineating boundaries for the country he pretended to rule. So vivid was Parodi's imagination that he created a constitution and passports for his domain.

Parodi's parents were unable to rein in their hyperactive son, so they banished him to Liceo Militar, a military school for difficult children. The top 10 students in the class were educated free of charge. Parodi's resentment of his father inspired him to study so that he would not have to seek financial assistance from him. Parodi's behavior also improved and he ranked second in his class during his final years. This was not the case for Parodi's younger brother, Roberto, who was expelled after 3 years. Roberto's record of 54 demerits for poor behavior stands today.

After graduation from Liceo Militar, Parodi enrolled at the University of Salvador in 1959. His most influential teachers were physicians, and Parodi excelled in biology, physiology, and physics. He worked nights as an operating room and emergency room assistant in order to maintain financial independence from his father. Although Parodi enjoyed internal medicine, he decided to become a surgeon in his fourth year at the University. Surgery suited his aggressive side and Parodi graduated in 1966 (Figure 24.1).

Parodi completed his surgical residency at the University of Buenos Aires in 1971. He desired a surgical residency with Rene Favaloro, an innovator of coronary bypass at the Cleveland Clinic, but no positions were available. Parodi went to the University of Illinois instead, at the invitation of Rudolph Mrazek. He spent 3 years there and transferred to the Cleveland Clinic when an opening became available in 1975. Parodi made the decision to become a vascular surgeon at the Cleveland Clinic, after extensive exposure to vascular trauma.

In 1976, Parodi returned to the University Hospital of Buenos Aires, where he remained on staff until 1983. It was during his first year there that Parodi con-

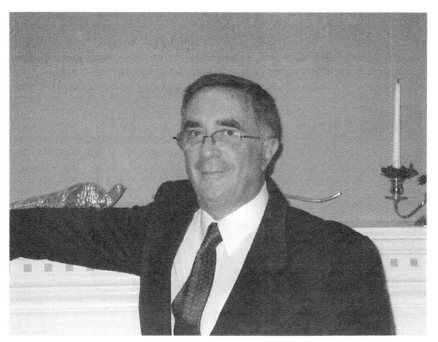

**Figure 24.1**  Juan Parodi, MD.

ceived the idea for endovascular repair of abdominal aortic aneurysms. Several consecutive patients had fared poorly after this operation, and Parodi pondered introduction of a prosthesis via the femoral arteries, thereby avoiding a laparotomy and retroperitoneal dissection. He devised a prototype in which a tube graft was pushed out of a plastic tube after it was advanced into the aneurysm; the system lacked a guidewire. When his single canine experiment failed, Parodi realized that a guidewire was essential, as was a retractable sheath.

Parodi was fortunate to have three brothers who were engineers: Guillermo was an industrial engineer, Roberto an agricultural engineer, and Carlos a mechanical engineer. Primarily with Carlos's assistance, and the help of his friend, Carlos Sommers, Parodi made numerous refinements of his endovascular graft, testing them all in dogs.

In 1978, Parodi married Graciela Suarez, after 6 years of courtship. They have two children, Julietta and Ezequiel, and a granddaughter, Augustina (Figures 24.2 and 24.3).

In 1983 Parodi left the University Hospital of Buenos Aires to begin the Instituto Cardiovascular de Buenos Aires. He was joined by Jorge Albertal, a cardiac surgeon trained at the Mayo Clinic; and Lardani Hector, a cardiologist from the Cleveland Clinic. Throughout this time, Parodi continued to tinker with his endovascular graft.

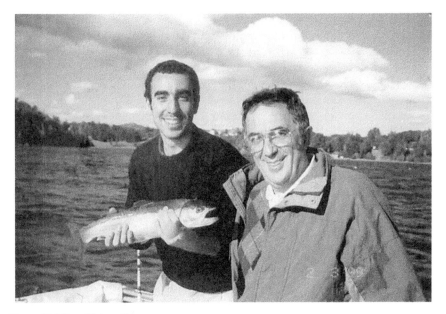

**Figure 24.2** Parodi leisure time.

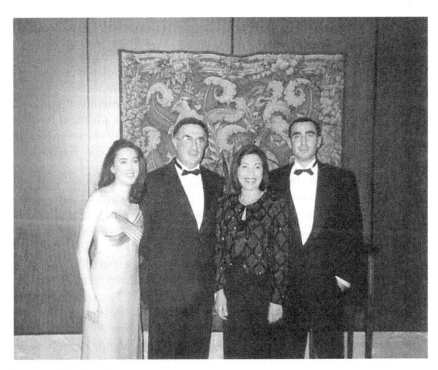

**Figure 24.3** The Parodi family.

In 1987, Parodi attended a lecture given by Juan Palmaz, describing the use of stents in animals. This gave him the idea for attaching stents to his endovascular grafts, rather than use a self-expanding system. Palmaz did not think it was a good idea.

With the continued assistance of Carlos Parodi and Carlos Sommer, Juan Parodi made a plastic abdominal aortic aneurysm model and tried his new system. Using new stents fashioned by Sommers at Citefa, a manufacturer of tanks and missiles, Parodi placed his grafts into 53 dogs with excellent results. Parodi personally financed all of his research and device manufacturing. He was now ready for the first clinical application of his graft.

Hector Coira was 75 years old in 1990. He was a farmer from outside Buenos Aires and suffered from severe chronic obstructive airway disease. He sought Parodi when he developed back pain from a large aneurysm. Parodi did not think Coira could survive a laparotomy, so he discussed his animal experiments with him. Parodi also met with Coira's brother and daughter to explain his new operation. On September 7, 1990, Parodi performed the first successful endovascular repair of an abdominal aortic aneurysm. The second aneurysm of the day required conversion to a laparotomy. On rounds that evening, Parodi was struck by the contrast between Coira sitting up in bed eating dinner, and his second patient intubated in the intensive care unit. Parodi reported his seminal case in an article entitled "Transfemoral Intraluminal Graft Implantation For Abdominal Aortic Aneurysms," in the *Annals Of Vascular Surgery*, in 1991. In the ensuing decade, thousands of patients throughout the world have benefited by Parodi's vision.

From 1993 through 1996 Parodi was Adjunct Associate Professor of Surgery at the Bowman Gray School of Medicine. Since 1998 he has been Professor of Surgery at the Wayne State University.

Parodi received the Jacobson Innovation Award of the American College of Surgeons in 1998. The following year he received the René Leriche Prize from the International Society of Surgery. The Honor Award for Excellence in Endovascular Surgery was bestowed upon Parodi by the International Society of Endovascular Specialists (ISES) in 2000.

Each year Parodi receives visitors from throughout the world at the Instituto Cardiovascular de Buenos Aires. More than 100 physicians are trained annually in all endovascular procedures. Parodi continues to perform almost 700 cases a year and is currently perfecting a cerebral protection device based upon reversal of flow in the internal carotid artery.

With a single idea, Juan Parodi transformed the practice of vascular surgery.

## Bibliography

Parodi JC, Palmaz JC, Barone HD. Transfemoral intraluminal graft implantation for abdominal aortic aneurysms. *Ann Vasc Surg* 1991; 5:491.

# Index

Printed and bound by CPI Group (UK) Ltd, Croydon, CR0 4YY

27/10/2024

14580190-0001